Tangled in the Curves

Real Life with Idiopathic Scoliosis

CAROLINE BELL

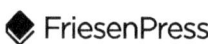

One Printers Way
Altona, MB R0G 0B0
Canada

www.friesenpress.com

Copyright © 2023 by Caroline Bell
First Edition — 2023

All rights reserved.

The information presented in this book is the author's opinion and personal experience. The content of this book is for general information purposes only and is not intended to diagnose, treat, cure, or prevent any condition or disease including scoliosis. It is not a substitute for professional medical advice, diagnosis, or treatment. Any information regarding medical conditions or treatments should be reviewed and discussed with a medical professional. Do not disregard or delay seeking professional medical advice due to the contents of this book.

No part of this publication may be reproduced in any form, or by any means, electronic or mechanical, including photocopying, recording, or any information browsing, storage, or retrieval system, without permission in writing from FriesenPress.

ISBN
978-1-03-917470-2 (Hardcover)
978-1-03-917469-6 (Paperback)
978-1-03-917471-9 (eBook)

HEALTH & FITNESS, DISEASES, MUSCULOSKELETAL

Distributed to the trade by The Ingram Book Company

To Mom and Dad, who continue to endure all of this with me.
Love always.

Preface

This book takes a look at life's little moments made extra special for those of us with moderate to severe scoliosis. Some things are trickier for us to figure out than for non-scoli people; other things come more naturally to us as we are treated to life lessons from "Professor Scoliosis." Sometimes it hurts; sometimes it doesn't. Sometimes the *ow* is physical; other times it's emotional. Sometimes we forget we have it; other times it's all we can think about. Most of all, at some point, scoliosis warriors can feel all alone in navigating it all, becoming tangled in the curves.

Do any of these sound familiar?

- I've just been diagnosed with scoliosis. What does that mean?
- Nobody else has felt this pain before.
- I don't know anybody with scoliosis. Should I talk to somebody else who has it?
- I don't want to talk about it.
- Is it normal that sitting a long time hurts?
- People won't understand what I'm feeling.
- What should I wear with my new brace?
- Standing too long hurts.
- Is therapy good for scoliosis? No physical therapy seems to be doing anything!
- What does life after spine surgery look like?
- I don't know what I should bring to the hospital to help with my recovery.
- What do I say to the school/office, if anything?
- Am I the only one who feels old and sore?
- My loved one has scoliosis, but I have no clue what that feels like or how to help. Where do I even start to gather information?
- Where can I find a more real-life perspective than the pamphlet the doctors gave me?

The short answer? Right here. This book wants to share with you the scoli life lessons many of us learned the hard way over the years. Knowing where to start and knowing other people have similar experiences can go a long way.

While researching for this book, I noticed some words scoliosis warriors associate with scoliosis: lonely, irritated, useless, annoyed, depressed, frustrated, in denial, stressed, tired, lost, anxious, helpless, hopeless, ashamed, motivated, scared, devastated, jealous, angry, overwhelmed, disappointed, sad, confused, defeated, misunderstood. What do these words all have in common? Aside from "motivated," they tell a pretty sad story. It's time for that narrative to change.

Let me very clearly reassure you that *you* are *not* alone. We are in fact a large and varied community of people who have tackled similar struggles in life due to scoliosis: soreness, imbalances, clothes, getting sad or mad, physical therapy, bracing, surgeries, too much information, not enough information, overly complicated information… We are resilient scoli warriors ready to support any newcomer in a warm embrace of our personal experiences, with a colossal mountain of tips and guidance at the ready. If you, yourself, do not have scoliosis, this book will give you a glimpse into what it's like living with a twisty spine and just how much warriors really earn their name.

Life is a series of choices, some of which you never imagined you'd need to make. Life is also a matter of perspective: glass half empty or glass half full? It's so easy to flip flop between choices and perspectives, dipping into the negative and pulling yourself back into the positive. Within these pages, I have tried to detail experiences with a realistic but supportive lens. Not all may apply to you, and you likely have additional experiences of your own. We are all different, after all – our spines, our minds, our situations, our families, our entire nervous systems.

You will never completely eradicate your idiopathic scoliosis, but with some time – and please be kind to yourself and give yourself that time – you can learn *from* it and how to best care *for* it.

Here are some key points to keep in mind:

1. You are not alone.

If you don't believe that at this moment, I encourage you to read on. You may be just another two-to-three-percent scoliosis statistic in the population, but those numbers add up to quite a warrior army.

This book was written with the intention of helping all scoliosis people understand they are not alone in dealing with the "quirks" of scoliosis. For those reading this who don't have scoliosis, hopefully this gives you a peek into what your loved ones or patients live with daily.

2. Every body is different.

All I know is what I've experienced. Your experiences are guaranteed to be unique, just as your curves are unique.

3. You are incredibly strong.

You can muster up more inner strength than you ever thought possible! This experience will make your amazing body and mind stronger, even though many times it may seem it is trying to break you down. You may even find yourself referring to your back in other tough situations, saying, "I've been through worse than this!"

4. Your shape has changed.

Your body is, in essence, being shifted by your own muscles and bones, which (as it sounds) can be uncomfortable. This can skew the center of gravity, move organs aside, and affect breathing. Things are different now.

5. Don't pretend it doesn't exist.

It *does* exist, and it needs your tender loving care.

6. Scoliosis-specific exercises and treatment exist.

Exercises can be catered to *your* back and its abilities or limitations. A therapist certified in Physiotherapy Scoliosis-Specific Exercises (PSSE) is trained to guide you in such exercise and education. Scoli- and fusion-friendly yoga, Pilates, stretching, and strengthening also exist. Invest in the right scoliosis education from a certified scoliosis professional for your unique back at the *beginning* of your journey as a solid building block.

7. Yeah, you could totally have done without it… but you can totally handle it.

We didn't ask for this, but some things you just can't change. I won't lie… there are rough spots. You may get frustrated and wonder, "Why me?"

Just go for a walk, go to scoli physio, speak to a psychologist, hug somebody, or simply do something fun! Move ahead with the good and keep learning. You have learned so much courtesy of your back – you may just not realize it yet.

8. You deserve to and *can* live a full life.

It may seem like scoliosis will stop you from leading a healthy, happy, normal life. With the perspective of experience, I can say with certainty *that is not the case*!

Your life is unique and absolutely does not need to be defined by scoliosis. You also have *nothing* to feel guilty about. There is so much more to life than your curves. Professor Scoliosis will be your teacher in self-care, self-acceptance, resilience, and determination.

9. Seek support. Talking about scoliosis helps.

Since I began my saga with scoliosis – which seems a lifetime ago – the internet has beefed up to offer tons of online and in-person scoliosis support groups and mentor programs for children, parents, and adults. Don't be shy to reach out and get involved. There are no extra points for going through this on your own. The emotional component cannot be ignored – more and more, psychology is recognized as a key support for scoliosis. Talking about it is far lighter than carrying it all alone!

Let's talk about what this book is *not*...

It is not a medical guide or specific exercise guide of any sort. That has to be left to the experts, which each scoli will need to seek out and learn from individually. I am an expert only in my own experiences and have corralled other warriors' expertise within their own unique scoli sagas. I've listed further reading and resources for specific expertise in the "Resources" section at the end of this book – I encourage you to continue your own research.

I hope you're able to use something from these pages to inspire your inner strength to surface. It may take hard work at times, but that does *not* mean it's impossible to handle. Ahead lies the good, the bad, and the ridiculous stuff we go through thanks to and in spite of scoliosis.

Thank you for joining me in this shared adventure.

Table of Contents

A Scoliosis Story 13
The Scoliosis Diagnosis 18
The Scoliosis Journey Before Surgery 20
    APPOINTMENTS 20
        Common terms and tools 20
        Doctor discussions 22
        Missing school/work for appointments 23
        That hospital smell 25
        The zen of X-rays 26
        Waiting in big hospital waiting rooms 27
        Waiting in little hospital examination rooms 27
    BRACING 29
        Back brace prescriptions 29
        Back brace adjustments 31
        Back brace accessories 32
        Back brace tips 33
        Staying warm during cold months 35
        The nighttime "shell waddle" 35
        Scoliosis at school 37
        Joking with your friends 38
    LESSONS AND REMINDERS 39
        Breathing 39
        Knowledge of your body 40
        It's not life-threatening 41
        You are not alone 42

The Scoliosis Journey for Surgery.. 43
   HOSPITAL TIME 43
      Setting the surgery date... 43
      Hospital prep... 44
      Operation day... 46
      Surgery séjour... 48
      Side-effects may include…... 51
      Pills and needles.. 53
      Sneezing 53
      Scars... 54
      Less curve, less prominence, less pain, more height 55
   HOME TIME 56
      Household prep 56
      Incentive spirometer 60
      The post-op poop... 60
      Re-learning basic life tasks 61
      Return-to-school prep.. 63
      No more regular radiation 64
      "Cured"? Okay, back to "normal" now!........................... 65

The Scoliosis Journey with a Fusion.. 67
   AROUND THE HOUSE 67
      Toilet paper dispenser location..................................... 67
      Bathtubs.. 68
      Making beds 69
      Gardening 70
      Wanting to stretch between your vertebrae 70
      Hot rod fevers 70
   OUT AND ABOUT 71
      Shoulder checking in cars 71

    Small cars = small door frames 71
    Vehicle seating 73
    Hardware science 74
    Spooky "new" pains 74
    Posture 75
    Classes at the gym 76
    Eating messy food at a low table 77
    Creating stories 77

The Scoliosis Journey Through Life 79

OW! WHAT A PAIN IN THE BACK 80
    Pain changes 80
    Pain is subjective 80
    Sitting for a long time 81
    Standing for a long time 83
    Horizontal for a long time 84
    Long days without stretching 85
    Stepping into a surprise dip in the ground 86
    The weird noises and cracks 87
    Feeling ancient 88
    These hips lie 89
    PMS: pretty mighty scoliosis 89
    Bad moods courtesy of pain 90
    Paingry 92
    Painsomnia 93
    Days with zero pain 94

MUST GET PHYSICAL 95
    Motion is lotion 95
    Going for walks 97
    Engage your core 98

Counter-stretching. All. The. Time.	99
Becoming an expert in your treatments	100

CONSIDERATIONS ... 105

Gravity	105
Money talks	105
Music	106
Scoliosis fashion	107
Need some inspiration?	108

NOT DESIGNED WITH YOU IN MIND ... 110

Hammocks	110
Hard chairs	110
Footwear	110
Kitchens	111
Babies	112

WISDOM AND STRENGTH ... 112

You are loved	112
Empathy	113
Surprising people	114
Responsibility	116
Deep appreciation for life	117
The power to help others	118

MIND AND MATTER ... 119

You know you have scoliosis	119
You know you're not exactly symmetrical	120
Hard on yourself	120
Repressing trauma	121
Beyond the physical	122
Crying	124
When you can't touch your toes	124

      Finally being able to touch your toes again 125
      Imagining what other people see 126
      Feeling normal most of the time 127
      You can get used to anything 128
  SCOLI INTERACTIONS 128
      People not understanding what scoliosis feels like 128
      Unsolicited advice 131
      Telling your new significant other 131
      A scoli in the wild! 132
  EXTERNAL FACTORS... 133
      The "idiopathic" in "idiopathic scoliosis" 133
      The genetic component 134
      Modern medicine... 134
      Internet research 136
      Media 138
  DEAR PARENTS, READ THIS 141
  THE BENEFITS OF POSITIVITY 145
Conclusion... 147
Acknowledgements 148
Resources 149
      Books 149
      Online learning... 150
      Physical and emotional support.. 151
      Research and education.. 152
      Scoliosis products 154
Endnotes... 155
Bibliography 160

A Scoliosis Story

Once upon a time, there was a girl who was of slim build and physically healthy. She was always the tallest girl in her grade, usually as tall or taller than most of the boys. In middle school, she started having pain in her neck and shoulders that no general-purpose medical professional could explain. Maybe it was the backpack? Maybe it was carrying too many textbooks? Likely just growing pains? Maybe it was too much activity? Not enough activity? Her family took her to physiotherapists, massage therapists, acupuncturists, and chiropractors to at least *try* and relieve the never-ending, tear-inducing, worsening pain. Nobody seemed to be able to explain it.

The summer she turned 15, she experienced a massive growth spurt – shot up to 5'10" within a matter of months. She spent that summer at a cottage on a lake swimming, tanning, running around, and having a grand ol' time. When school started back up that fall, she was tall, bleach blonde, and bronzed. She was excited to make new friends, join clubs, and create high school memories. In her first months of that school year, she thrived despite continued shoulder pain and a new back pain. Overall, it appeared life was going according to plan.

As it turns out, there was another plan afoot, waiting to reveal itself. One day that fall, as she was heading out to the bus stop, her father gave her a hug and when his arms went around her back, he froze and said, "Wait… what's that? Turn around for a second." Lo and behold, a mass of muscle had built up on the left side of her lower back and her opposite shoulder blade was poking out. What the heck was that? Had she run into something? Did she sleep wrong? She had been seeing a chiropractor every week for months. If it was anything bad, surely they would have caught it…

Off to the family doctor they went.

Within mere minutes, the doc knew what it was: adolescent idiopathic scoliosis (AIS). It had developed over a few months and none of the professionals had noticed it. Two curves (around 30 and 50 degrees) were present.

The next order of business was to head back to the chiropractor's office. A tense but brief conversation ensued about why the heck they'd been saying "everything looks good" for the last few months; how they could have missed something this big, knowing full well it was in the family tree; and what exactly they thought they were being paid for all this time when she was still in pain. (Note: This chiropractor does not represent the quality of all chiropractors.)

Then came the flurry of hospital appointments, X-rays, and orthotist fittings for a back brace.

In case you haven't caught on by this point, I was that girl. My initial reaction was quite lackluster, to be honest. "Oh. Okay. Well, a couple of women in my family have it and they do everything just fine. And it isn't hurting much more than before, so... Can I go home now, doctor?" My parents, being adults, were understandably more educated and aware of the situation and its possible outcomes.

Thus began an entire new chapter in my life, which was not without its own challenges. Little did I know it was just the beginning. I wished so much everything would stay the same and, like those couple of women in my family, it would have little impact on my life. But if that were the case, I'd have nothing to fill these pages with, now would I? And more importantly, I would not have lived through the experiences – all before I could legally vote or drive – that made me the strong person I am today. Feeling all alone with scoliosis seemed to steal pieces of my youth, but it also set me up with a lifetime of resilience and determination.

Following diagnosis, the next challenge presented itself in the form of a nighttime back brace. The goal was to try and slow down those two curves as I continued to grow. When those curves showed no intention of slowing down – seemingly fully committed to being scoliotic – I made the very difficult decision at 17 years old to undergo spinal fusion surgery (which is exactly what it sounds like). In the simplest terms, that day changed my life. It was the biggest test I never expected to face.

As I flitted through life with scoliosis, pre-fusion and post-fusion, I occasionally kept a daily tally of the number of times I uttered the sound "*ow*." On average, *ow* came out of my mouth 10 times a day. And sure, some of those were from running into coffee tables, suffering paper cuts, stepping on rocks, or being stung by bugs. But the majority happened just because I *moved*.

We're not talking Olympic-style feats here. No running, jumping, falling, diving, or flipping. Just your average, run-of-the-mill, going-about-your-day movements:

- Standing up from the couch: "*ow*"
- Reaching for the top-shelf cookies: "*ow*"
- Getting in or out of a car: "*ow*"
- Sitting for too long: "*ow*"
- Spending a day slowly walking through a museum: "*ow*"
- Reaching down to tie my shoes too quickly: "*ow*"
- Picking up a box and forgetting to engage my core: "*ow*"

I lived in near-constant pain with no long-term plan, only short-term relief from never-ending general-purpose physical therapists that didn't consider or address my unique spine. I poured buckets of time, effort, and money into exercises designed for a "non-scoli" back for years, sometimes causing more harm than good. I was limited to interactions with therapists who didn't know much about scoliosis or with doctors who were focused solely on talking clinical details and X-rays, never mind the scoliosis effects of pain and imbalances on *life*.

I erroneously believed that because my spine was curved, it made me different and therefore I needed to hide away. I would opt out of certain outfits for fear of "it" showing or decline plans with friends in case something would hurt. My back was an influential factor in my life… and not in a healthy way. It didn't help that, as far as I knew, I was the only person dealing with a spine as curvy, painful, and surgically enhanced as mine. I kept my head down, my eyes shut, my emergency pain meds at hand, and hunkered down for a life peppered with gloomy days. Sore and alone without a fool-proof treatment plan, the future was a scary unknown.

For over a decade I was under the impression that I was a solo act in the world of scoliosis management. That feeling of being all alone started when I got my diagnosis and went on for 15 years until I finally stopped being angry and started being inquisitive. I joined online scoliosis communities, eventually meeting with other "fusioneers."

I had very low expectations that life could be different from what I had known, but still, I set an initial goal to exchange support, guidance, and encouragement with fellow "scoliosis warriors." Imagine my shock when I was reassured that I was not "doomed" to live in pain forever, did not need to hide, and most importantly was not alone. I was equally stunned at the number of adults speaking openly about their experience for the first time *ever*, overwhelmed with emotion, saying things like, "Finally, somebody who actually understands what it feels like. All these years, *I thought it was just me.*"

These communities revealed something else as well. I was saddened at the number of families just like mine desperately seeking the *same* answers to the *same* questions and fears about diagnosis, bracing, surgery, and pain that we had had ages ago. Here was a symphony of folks who also believed they were on their own, holding on to a sliver of hope that things could be better.

Now that some time has passed since my bracing and surgery (allowing me to gain perspective around it all), it feels like the perfect time to examine the full scoliosis journey and its effect on so many lives. Back in the 2000s, support material was pretty much nonexistent, with the few resources available being negative, medical, and far too complicated. I had no idea if what I was going through was "normal," what to wear under my brace, if surgery was the right choice, what was involved in surgical recovery, and what the rest of my day-to-day-life would be like. I was terrified of the unknown, and rightfully so. The internet was around, but it certainly was not as bountiful as it is today. It's still tricky to find correct, relevant, evidence-based information in this sea of content, but even trickier is the new rule of thumb for the modern era: Don't believe everything you read on the internet.

I wanted to create something that spoke solely and honestly to the scoliosis experience, which you, dear reader, may be living. In the hopes of giving you as many plain-language perspectives and as much guidance as possible, I have dug into scientific research, sought expert insight, and compiled scoliosis warrior stories and tips from around the globe, including anecdotes from my own personal journey. It's what I would have wanted to read in support of my scoliosis journey through each stage. I am moved beyond words by the eagerness of other scoliosis warriors to share their experiences and education – across decades and continents – to help their scoliosis community – thank you all!

This book is a contribution to making information about the scoliosis experience centrally and readily available from a "real person" perspective – a point of view rarely handed over at the doctor's office. The heart-wrenching realization that families are still not being given real-life information to kick-start their scoli saga and that long-term scoli-endurers are still *hiding in pain sight* without bountiful support led me to sit down and write this book. Through these pages, I aim to give scoli young adults, scoli elders, scoli parents, and scoli caregivers insights, ideas, and support throughout this scoliosis journey that none of us asked for.

The Scoliosis Diagnosis

Let's begin here: What is this scoliosis thing? It's certainly not something you hear in everyday conversation or see regularly on the evening news. Scoliosis is a medical condition where the spine's vertebrae *bend, curve,* and *rotate* in all three dimensions.[1] To be diagnosed with scoliosis, the left-to-right (or "coronal") curvature has to have at least a 10-degree Cobb angle (a standard measurement used to measure a spine's curve). This happens in roughly two to three percent of people around the world.[2] An estimated seven million people in the United States alone have scoliosis.[3] Keeping in mind that scoliosis affects people globally, that adds up to a great army of scoliosis warriors! Interestingly enough, the World Health Organization website has no mention of scoliosis.[4]

Many people with scoliosis live pain-free and require no treatment, but many others are in regular discomfort or even pain. Every single body and mind is different, and we all experience the condition uniquely. Some people have one curve at the top of the spine. Others have one at the bottom. Some get a combo of two or three curves. Every curve is unique in location, size (curvature degree), rotation, and effect on neighboring body parts, like hips and shoulders. Scoliosis has a three-dimensional impact, not just a side-to-side bend. Scoliosis does not care who you are, where you're from, or how intelligent you may be. It can just show up without any explanation about its origins or how curvy and rotated it plans to get.

There are many different treatment types out there, but bracing and surgery are in the spotlight. An estimated 30,000 children in the United States are prescribed braces each year.[5] There are many different brace models available as well, and the requirements – day or night, number of hours, number of years – are unique to each patient. As for surgery, spinal fusions are not exclusively for scoliosis. In 2018, spinal fusions were the sixth most common operating room procedure for inpatient stays and the most expensive procedure, with up to $14.1 billion in costs.[6]

In addition to bracing and surgery, there are scoliosis physical therapies available that can help, whether the spine is fused or not. Below are seven different schools that use PSSE concepts which have shown excellent results in addressing curvatures and alignments. Any of these approaches could be included in a treatment plan:

- Lyon approach from France
- Schroth method from Germany
- Scientific Exercise Approach to Scoliosis (SEAS) from Italy
- Barcelona Scoliosis Physical Therapy School (BSPTS) from Spain
- DoboMed approach from Poland
- Side Shift method from the United Kingdom
- Functional Individual Therapy of Scoliosis (FITS) method from Poland

A whopping 80 percent of all scoliosis cases are diagnosed as idiopathic scoliosis.[7] Adolescent idiopathic scoliosis includes "adolescent" because people tend to develop this type of scoliosis between the ages of 10 and 15[8]; "idiopathic" means there is no definite cause. Idiopathic scoliosis appears to affect girls eight times more often than boys,[9] and a lot of research is looking into a potential genetic contribution from the family tree. Scoliosis affects much more than just the physical side, however, and the importance of adolescent warriors having strong emotional support is finally beginning to surface.[10]

It can feel overwhelming to be given buckets of information mere moments after a receiving diagnosis of scoliosis. If you don't remember it all right away, that's okay. If you don't feel like you know what to do right now, that's okay. If you're scared and feel like your world just shrank to the size of a marble, that's okay.

Receiving a diagnosis of scoliosis can be an emotional time full of questions and concerns. Don't forget to take a step back to breathe instead of trying to drink from the firehose. We'll get into much more information throughout this book, which you can read at your own pace and refer to whenever you feel like it. There is no time limit and no stress of a doctor's office here.

The Scoliosis Journey Before Surgery

Are you freshly diagnosed, in a brace, or living with some non-surgically-reinforced natural curves? This section covers explanations, tips, and lessons learned during the next chapter of scoli life. The learning doesn't stop throughout scoli life, but it can certainly feel like there's a lot more to absorb at the beginning. You'll notice your physical and emotional scoli situations are not isolated to your world – many of us run into challenges and lessons through these phases.

If you're just starting out, hopefully this can give you a "heads up." If you're in it now, maybe you can find some comfort knowing we went through it too. If you're many years past the early stages but these experiences come back in a flash of memory, I hope you can make peace with them and move on from those days. Maybe they can serve as reminders of all you've learned.

Here is what real life with scoliosis before or without spinal fusion surgery can look like and feel like.

APPOINTMENTS

Common terms and tools

After a few appointments, you will begin to recognize some common terms and tools around scoliosis doctors' offices. Expect your height and weight to be measured every time, along with the many degrees along your spine. Also expect to do "Adam's forward bend test" over and over again, bending forward to touch your toes for a minute or so while somebody looks at your back.[11] You will run into a little tool called a "scoliometer," which is essentially a plastic level used to measure the rotation of the spine or "angle of trunk rotation."[12] These often go hand in hand with early detection testing.

You will learn about the sections of the spine. From top to bottom: cervical, thoracic, lumbar, and sacrum. Your doctor should have a spine model somewhere in the office, and they should review with you where your scoliosis curves are located. At the same time, they can explain the significance of the "lordosis" and "kyphosis" curves in your spine – which you can see when standing with your side to a mirror.[13] Scoliosis is three dimensional and does not affect the spine only in one side-to-side direction, after all.[14]

X-rays will be taken to measure the spine's curvature in degrees known as Cobb angles; these are the curves traditionally shown in X-ray pictures on websites and social media with little triangular lines drawn across them. Pay attention in your math class, because the Cobb angle is about numbers. They take the top of your curve, the bottom of your curve, draw some lines to make a triangle, add in some math, and that's how doctors get what "degree" your curves are. Depending on the number of curves in the spine, there could be more than one angle to report on.[15]

You'll hear about "Risser" and "Sanders" numbers.[16] These represent phases of ossification (bone growth) that indicate how much growing remains. The Risser number comes from an X-ray of growth plates in the pelvis (which is captured during spine X-rays), while the Sanders number comes from X-rays of the hand. This information influences bracing and surgery decisions.

Through all of this, it will be important to know your Cobb angles and curve locations, but also where your "concavities" and "convexities" are. These are the parts of your torso that are essentially larger or smaller, due to the curve and rotation of the spine. Your PSSE therapist can give you all the information you want and more about this important topic, including an explanation of how scoliosis is three-dimensional and not just about your Cobb angles.

You may also be checked for something called "Marfan syndrome" and "generalized joint hypermobility," both of which can be related to scoliosis. Depending on your overall health and whether or not you're preparing for surgery, you may be sent for blood work. Girls, be warned that doctors are particularly interested in your iron levels.

Some at-home tools include heating pads, ice packs, and exercise balls of all sizes. Those can come in very handy! There are also all kinds of pain-reducing creams and gels on the market to try out. Over-the-counter pain meds can take the ache out of a tired lower back or stressed shoulder being pushed around by scoliosis.

Doctor discussions

Medicine is a great big world of information and terminology. Do *not* take it personally if you don't understand everything the medical professionals say about your back right away. You are not supposed to know every detail, term, rationale, and treatment plan. You are young, and also *you are not a doctor*. If you find yourself feeling lost, try and recognize it and then give yourself a break.

This may be the very beginning of your scoliosis journey. As with every new beginning, there is a whole new world of information you cannot instantly know and understand. The learning is not going to stop, but it does need to start. One step at a time. Even though you don't know the name of every vertebra, muscle, tendon, and ligament in your back, you *do* know that you have a spine. Excellent start! Now let's get familiar with the sections of the back: "cervical" (neck region), "thoracic" (chest region), and "lumbar" (lower back region). Next up: Where are your curves? What a great intro conversation to have with your doctor. You're going to *want* to know this and you *need* to know this, so have a chit-chat with your professional, ask questions, and don't be shy about asking for clarification if what they say doesn't make sense to you.

Remember that your professionals want to help you and certainly want you to be well informed. At the same time, not every surgical pro is a medical genius *and* a warm teddy bear. Some of these medics are *extremely* intelligent and that doesn't always translate well into explaining things simply. They're so knowledgeable that it can seem dirt simple to them while being brand new and complicated to you. It is the care team's responsibility to recommend the best medical options to support your physical health, but they also need to empathize, listen, build trust, and explain complicated things in ways you and your family will understand.[17] Care teams need to be patient-focused and not just illness-focused.[18] The teams should no longer simply burst in with medical tests and doctor vernacular: "How many hours did you wear your brace? Did you do your exercises every day? Here are your current Cobb angles." Know that there *are* doctors out there who are well versed in both aspects – medical and emotional.

The medical and emotional combo can be a lot for a few team members to learn and manage. You can help by focusing on your side of this equation and becoming a member of the team. Write out questions you have about your health *in advance* of your appointment to build up your own knowledge base. Add in specifics about how you feel on certain days to give you something to springboard off of when you're in a meeting with them in case you're a bit anxious or shy. Ask them for written details of what was discussed at the appointment so you can re-read it at home when you're in a calmer state of mind.[19]

You may also run into professionals who inspect your back but mainly address your parents or caregivers in the room. This one can be annoying. After all, it's your back, your body, and your health, so why wouldn't the medical team be addressing *you*? You're not just the vessel for the discussion at hand, here! Maybe they thought leaving you out of the heavy conversations would make it easier on you, or maybe the professional is just more comfortable speaking to adult parents who may "understand it more."

In the meantime, you're going to have to speak up if this is bothering you. Nobody can guess what you're feeling or thinking; you have to use your voice to ask questions, seek clarifications, and include yourself in discussions about *your* health. Talk with your caregivers about what you need: Would you prefer the doctors speak with your caregivers separately about some topics, or would you prefer the doctors have direct conversations with you about all details? This is where you learn the importance of advocating for yourself – clearly communicate what you need for your health.

Missing school/work for appointments

Most scoliosis diagnoses occur during puberty as they're often partnered with growth spurts.[20] (Remember the A in AIS stands for "adolescent.") This means this fun rollercoaster is likely to start while in middle school or high school, a time already loaded with social pressures and self-esteem battles. A scoliosis diagnosis also comes with a lot of appointments: specialists, X-rays, hospitals, back brace adjustments, physiotherapy, massage therapy... All of these take up time.

Since evenings are not always an option, sometimes these appointments have to happen in the middle of the day (during regular doctor working hours). And hospitals can't always give you the luxury of selecting your appointment time as they are swamped with tons of patients and hindered by limited resources. You take what you're given.

Know what this means? You get to dip out of class early or miss some boring school assembly. Just consider it a perk and enjoy it! A few non-standard agenda days are a nice break from the daily humdrum of school. Something going on in the real world on a Tuesday morning outside of school? Cool! Maybe your caregivers take you for lunch afterwards. It's really not that bad of a deal, all things considered.

It does, however, come with some planning requirements. For starters, high school classes are relatively small. Being with the same circle of classmates day in and day out, you become aware of each other's habits and definitely notice when someone is absent. Especially if they are absent a lot. I was often absent for doctors' appointments and endured a few sideways comments of the "she was away again yesterday, what's wrong with her" flavor. But I was lucky in the high school lottery with extremely supportive friends and teachers. They would inquire as to my whereabouts to make sure I was okay and, for the most part, I left it at "doctor's appointment." It is entirely up to you how much detail you decide to tell people. Just know that people are bound to notice your absences, and piles of white lies can be exhausting.

Aside from the social aspect, education may also take a bit of a hit. Being away from class means missed lessons, missed assignments, and sometimes missed tests. It helps to be honest with the teacher as soon as you find out you have a non-negotiable appointment coming up that will take you out of class. Go see them during lunch, respectfully give them a heads up, and ask if you can have the lesson notes in advance. Alternative accommodations for tests can also be coordinated. Yes, it's a bit more of a hassle, but remember that you're dealing with mature adults here. The teachers want what's best for your education, and this flows right into college. Thankfully your college schedule provides more daytime slots for appointments, making this whole scoliosis scheduling thing way easier.

If you're hoping scoliosis will just go away on its own and your spine will straighten out without any help... let me tell you *hope* is not a great strategy here. Appointments are being booked for a reason, and you should take every one of them seriously.

Let's jump into the post-secondary world of work. You work for and with adults. You know how appointments work by now and everybody should be grown-up about it. It becomes a bummer when requesting time off is complicated or you have a limited amount offered to you. Give your supervisor plenty of notice, and plan as much as possible to take your appointments outside of work hours. Just do your best... as always.

That hospital smell

I don't know how they do it, but hospitals (much like casinos) seem to have one standard odor no matter where you go. It's a special blend of industrial cleaning products, forced air, and sadness... also not unlike a casino. The only thing missing is the aroma of cigarettes. Hospitals are, of course, not perfume departments nor do they have any requirement to maintain a pleasant-smelling garden aroma; they're supposed to be as sterile as possible while on a budget. Let's also acknowledge that many people have serious perfume allergies.

Yet somehow that "hospital smell" sent butterflies through my tummy for years. I found myself wondering, "Why can't it be improved?" My mother had high hopes of me growing up to be a nurse when I was a little girl. Those dreams promptly went out the window when, after a few too many bad-news visits, I began feeling instantly lightheaded whenever I walked through the front hospital doors. Deep breaths and self-reassurance were needed throughout in spades. Isn't it ironic that hospitals can feel so *inhospitable*? Thankfully, as the bad-news visits tapered off, the butterflies seemed to fly away.

It certainly doesn't help that *smell* is the oldest sense. Even better, the part of your brain that directly handles all scents that enter your snoot, the olfactory bulb, happens to be right beside the part of your brain that creates new memories, the hippocampus.[21] When you also consider that there are at least 1,000 different scent receptor types deeply connected to your brain, it's no wonder that scents can trigger memories and feelings.[22] Even if you can't quite put them into words, those scent memories are very real. There's a lot of fascinating research into this neuroscience topic that isn't "scary" to read, if you want to do some research of your own.

The zen of X-rays

The waiting game becomes familiar after a while, especially when you end up visiting the *waiting* room regularly. It becomes a kind of trance when you walk across that threshold: You cue up the X-ray appointment zen mode. You have nowhere else to be right now, so just give in to the extended waiting time you will spend here and turn off your brain. Nothing bad or painful will happen to you in this place.

Allow me to paint you a picture: You're sitting in a bright waiting room. It's quiet except for the air vents humming, fluorescent lights whining, and front desk receptionist fielding non-stop calls. There are other people sitting around you, some on their own and others with a partner or parent. You're all sitting in mysteriously uncomfortable chairs in a place where most folks are broken one way or another. Dog-eared magazines are lying around on tables and chairs, waiting to serve as time-killers once again.

Finally, the technician walks into the room; all eyes immediately turn to her with hope that they'll be chosen next. She says your name – you're the winner of this round! You follow her into a tiny hallway (it's never a grand hall back there) lined with change rooms. She tells you that same rehearsed line: "Everything off, including your bra. You can keep your socks and underwear. Gown open in the back. Open the curtain when you're done and I'll come get you."

Pro tip: If there isn't a stack of gowns in the change room, you can ask for a second one if you have more appointments in the building that day and have been instructed to remain in this gown for the duration. Put the second gown opening in the front so that your bum won't moon anybody in the hallways. Plus, it's warmer in that cool hospital air. If they don't have more or you're too shy to ask, pack a long sweater that day – use that as your stylish "second gown."

So, you change into the gown(s) and open the curtain to your change room. The technician comes over and leads you to the X-ray room. It's dark and cool in there. You're alone with the technician and time slows: no clocks, no windows, no sense of hurry, just weird machines with blinking lights… like a casino except nobody wins. Just take a deep breath and go through the motions. *Ahhhh* zen.

She'll ask you to stand in front of a screen, lie on a table, or step into an EOS imaging machine depending on what the doctor ordered. EOS imaging machines, by the way, have the easiest X-ray process I've ever seen. It's like walking into a metal-detector machine at the airport, where you just step into a box for a moment, lift up your arms, something happens around you with you barely noticing, and then you walk out. The bonus is that these have far lower radiation levels than traditional X-rays, which is good to consider if you're going to be getting regular X-rays for your scoliosis.[23]

Deep breath, hold it, click-click, done. Then maybe a quick X-ray of your hand to capture some growth indicators. And that's it! Back to the change room, back to the waiting room, and on to the day's next order of business. Maybe even a stop for ice cream on the way home?

What a nice break from the monotony of a usual day, with a lack of bad news and an abundance of zen!

Waiting in big hospital waiting rooms

If you haven't yet experienced enough of these to know they have their own aura, then trust me when I say you will. The waiting time and silence in-between appointments becomes its own time-halting saga during a fun hospital day.

The anticipation builds up. You wait. You stress. You see other kids around you too, knowing they're also there due to some health issue. Your family waits with you since you're likely a preteen and can't drive yourself. You watch your loved ones eagerly await some news.

Hark! They call your name on the speaker system! Oh, great. Everybody there now knows your name… Never mind them! You're all there for the same reason.

Get your stuff, lead the way, move from one waiting room to another, and get comfy for the next portion of your day: the little hospital examination room.

Waiting in little hospital examination rooms

Waiting room vibe, intensified. Like nearing the peak of the story arc in a Hollywood movie. This whole day has led up to this. "What's gonna happen? Anything could happen!" Anticipation and hope mix together, paired with (probably) too much sitting. Any news is big news. Come on! Why are they running late again?

You can hear the ceiling lights buzzing and some muted conversations from the hallways and neighboring rooms. Hopefully some good news is being delivered nearby.

Waiting, waiting, waiting.

"Everything is so sanitary. Why are all of these rooms always white? The lighting is super fluorescent and synthetic. How about something happy painted on the walls instead? Maybe make it look less like a 'hospital' scene. Everybody is already stressed out being here. How about a nice calm blue or earthy green? I wonder what they keep in those cupboards. What the heck is the point of paper on the examination bed? How many people have received good news in here? Bad news? Likely a bit of both. My goodness, this has been way too much alone time with my thoughts, today!"

You've paired your worries with your parents' worries – you're feeding off of each other's eagerness to find out the updates in your health portfolio. Such suspense! Cue the typical dad, swooping in to lighten the mood. He tries out the blood pressure machine because he's either curious, bored, trying to entertain you, trying to embarrass you, or trying to think of anything other than the news about to come in through the door. (Or all of the above.)

Ah, here we go! A resident doctor appears to ask some preliminary questions and maybe conduct a quick physical assessment – they're in training and you're a great example of scoliosis, after all. This will be an easy examination, since you're probably still sporting that drab hospital gown from your X-rays three hours ago. If you prefer to have the examination without your parents around, say so. (Doctors should offer this anyway.)

The resident leaves to mumble a conversation with the doctor in the hall. Finally, your doctor appears! The grand finale of the day! Let's hope it begins with some nice small talk about life and non-scoliosis stuff. Then a quick recap of the previous X-rays versus the latest ones, a second back examination, feedback on the brace's effectiveness (if applicable), and suggested next steps. If the doctor doesn't provide you a written summary about what you all talked about today, ask for something in writing.

BRACING

Back brace prescriptions

If you've just been diagnosed with scoliosis, you may be prescribed a brace. This corrective device has been deemed the best route to take by the healthcare experts monitoring your health. Trust that your doctors are prescribing a brace for a *reason* and not just for fun.

Have you ever seen a tall plant in a garden start growing over to one side? Sometimes that plant just needs a couple of supports, like sticks, to help it grow straighter. Back braces are kind of like those supports. Many people have had back braces, and many of them have had corrective results. Sure, there are annoying things about braces (which this book only touches on), but in the grand scheme of life (a) your body is your home and you have to care for it, (b) you're not going to see most people from high school ever again and any external opinions of your brace are insignificant in comparison to your health, (c) a few months in a brace out of 90 years of life is a tiny blip in your timeline, and (d) early bracing is an opportunity to improve spine alignment, likely in combination with some physical exercises. It may not be the highlight of your life, but it also may not be the worst thing. Surgery is not the end of the world, should it be required, but it has more risks than this little cocoon. Do the best you can with your brace and take it seriously.

There are tons of medical corrective devices out there other than back braces, as you know. Look around and you'll see hearing aids and eyeglasses. Their purposes are similar yet different. After all, a hearing aid doesn't improve someone's hearing to the point they no longer need that corrective device – hearing aids are long-term. Do you see the silver lining here? Back braces are *temporary*, and your young spine is still flexible enough to change.

There have been numerous brace designs over the years with all kinds of materials, styles, and success rates: Milwaukee brace, Charleston bending brace, Wilmington brace, Wood Chêneau Rigo (WCR) brace, SpineCor brace, Whisper brace... Thankfully we have moved away from metal on to plastics. Designers have even trimmed down the thickness of the material and padding required while maintaining success rates. This is important to keep in mind – the lightest, thinnest brace is of no use if it isn't actively correcting the curves and rotations. There are massive implications of not doing a good job at the bracing stage. Good bracing specialists will be hesitant to jump on board with the next big thing making a splash in the world of scoliosis bracing until solid data can be presented. Many new brace designs have surfaced over the last decade, finally taking into consideration the 3-D aspect of scoliosis and using that to its advantage.[24]

The process of creating a brace has also progressed over the years. When I was fitted for my brace, it took two people about an hour to wrap me in layers of plaster-soaked strips. It felt like I was being turned into a piñata, but sadly no candy was involved. It wasn't painful, more of a nuisance and an exercise in patience. Today, technology strikes again. While that "piñata" molding is still used, brace designs can now be drafted using scanners, tablets, and computers. This makes it extra easy on the patient and brace fitter. Designs may be sent offsite to be fabricated or made in-house; the patient may even get to help out or watch. You don't get to choose the specific shape of the brace, but you do get to pick the brace's color design. Orthotists – the people who make braces – have tons of patterns and colors to choose from. They also do the assessment and have the vision to create the perfect brace for each unique patient – it's science and art. Adjustments are made in-house, an X-ray is taken while wearing the brace, and the rest is up to the patient to take their brace schedule seriously.

You have to trust that those around you want what's best, have faith that *you* are doing the right thing in caring for *you*, and hang on to that inner strength... as tough as it may seem some days. Don't stop doing the things you love to do! Keep your friends and family close, and talk about your brace if you're having a frustrating moment with it.[25] You don't have to do it on your own.

> **Dear Parents:** Choosing a brace type during a diagnosis stage can seem overwhelming. There is a *lot* of information to go through in the short amount of time between diagnosis and meeting with a brace fitter. Take your time as much as possible to read up on different brace types and success rates. Do *not* grab the first brace to cross your path – remember that some people are better salespeople than others, and some are experts in only one type, which is what they'll promote. If unsure where to start, check out one of the many resources listed at the end of this book.

Back brace adjustments

Know this: It won't fit perfectly right off the bat. Let's set realistic expectations that the first few days in a back brace are going to be tough but that it only gets easier from there. The brace fitter knows it will need some adjusting; in fact, they plan it in as part of your additional visits. It's the same deal as with any orthodontics or new shoes: You have to break it in.

After your measurements, X-rays, and prescription have been turned into an actual brace, you get to try it on at the orthotist's office. These experts will know what needs adjusting right off the bat just by seeing you in it. They may have you put it on and take it off a few times as they adjust it here and there using special tools to trim, shave, and melt it. They may also send you home with it for a night to see how sleeping goes and schedule a follow-up visit for additional adjustments. They'll also need to take some X-rays while you're wearing the brace to make sure it's correcting the curves properly. All this to say: You will have more than one visit with them.

Complete and total comfort may be a lost cause here, but it shouldn't *hurt* you. If you're experiencing immense pain, or if your brace is moving around so much that it's creating blisters, your brace likely needs to be adjusted. Mine was crushing a small section of my front rib cage that protruded from my spinal rotation. It hurt so badly that it was waking me up at night – I knew something wasn't right so I booked another adjustment visit. Calmly and explicitly tell your orthotist what you're feeling and where it hurts. Be clear that it's keeping you up at night just because of one spot and is otherwise as comfortable as it can be. Could they cut or melt one part open to give two ribs some breathing room? The team tackles many puzzles and likely has some ideas of how to improve it for you.

It bears mentioning that these are professionals who make braces and orthotics to *help* people. They know what they're doing and they're trying to improve your health by creating a custom piece of equipment. You may be going through a lot of stress, but don't take it out on them.

Once you take your shiny new brace home, you'll be given a schedule to slowly get into the feel and habit of it (usually a few hours at a time). Regardless of whether it's a day or night brace, you're not going to pop this thing on and go on with your regular program. It's a big, strong tool that needs some getting used to. I'll admit that I cried the first couple of weeks before it was completely adjusted, since it needed more padding and tweaks, and I hadn't yet perfected my outfits. Heads up that your skin may temporarily turn a bit red as it gets used to this new brace. One simple thing you can avoid is body lotion – softer skin can become irritated more easily.

Don't expect to figure it all out right away... nobody does. This is something that takes time and practice, with some trial-and-error moments for bending and moving. Give yourself permission to take this experience one moment at a time.

Back brace accessories

Should you be prescribed a back brace, it will send you on a quest for new brace-friendly clothing. We all go on that mission – driving all around town, scouring every store, trying to find clothes to wear *under* the brace and *over* the brace, buying them, trying them on at home, returning them – as we try to figure out this new plastic cocoon. Every brace is as unique as every person; clothing is personal to each individual and brace.

My night brace was so tight and padded that anything with a thick seam or wrinkle would be carved into my skin by morning – sometimes, in the early days, even waking me up in pain. My mother (God bless her) and I went on a mission. It took a while – as does every brace mission in the beginning – until we found something that matched my comfort needs. We eventually found at a department store a super-thin cami and tight t-shirt with thin seams along the sides. We took them home to try out for the night along with a pair of boy's boxer shorts with a wide, flat elastic waistband. Those three items worked so well we went back and bought every color available! If you have a day brace, don't be shy about doing the same thing; you can even make it a semi-annual event to load up on under-brace clothes. When it works, it works!

While shopping missions are still a part of the brace experience, thankfully fellow scoliosis warriors have taken it upon themselves to design brace-specific undershirts to make your life easier. (You'll find useful links in the "Resources" section at the end of this book.) These undershirts are very long so the top edge can fold down over the upper rim of a brace, giving the impression of a tank top while softening hard brace edges under the armpits. Of course, you're welcome to shop off the rack; make sure to check out all sections (boys, girls, and gender-neutral)... whatever works! But count your lucky stars that such brace-specific accessories are now available to you without the need to drive all around town. If you have specific parts of the brace rubbing or pushing against you (under the armpit is a popular spot), consider sewing your own little cloth cover for that section to soften it against your skin. Just check with your orthotist first to make sure it's permitted.

What about brace transportation? You can keep it loose, but you now also have the option of using specially designed bags for back braces. These are definitely tougher and cuter brace containers than the black garbage bag I had to use back in the day. What a superior way to keep your brace close by and well protected on a plane, train, road trip, or just for storing it during soccer practice. Give your hard-working brace some TLC! It may even provide an opportunity for educational conversation to help those who are uncomfortable about it, boosting self-confidence throughout.

If you wear a brace at night, sleeping flat on your back can make you feel like a vulnerable turtle. Sleeping on your stomach is equally difficult to flip yourself over. Sleeping on the side flops you forward or backward if there's nothing there to support you... so let's add in that support! Invest in a body or maternity pillow. Adjust it however you need to create a comfortable and safe nest. You can also toss your arms around this pillow instead of them falling asleep from being pinned under your shell.

Back brace tips

Time to make life with back braces easier. Ready? Begin!

While I only have firsthand experience with nighttime braces, speaking with full-time "bracers" (those who wear braces) has revealed that the following is true of all braces: They're hot. They restrict movement. They're not exciting to put on. They'll require time to master accompanying outfits. And yet, you *will* figure it all out.

Let's talk about brace tips, starting with hot nights: Do *not* wear your birthday suit under it, even if you think "less clothes will be less hot." You will stick and rub against it, potentially causing blisters. You will need to go on a mission to find soft fabric that breathes (preferably moisture-wicking) and wear that underneath no matter what the mercury says. As mentioned, be careful about seams and wrinkles that dig into your skin.

If the weather where you live gets quite hot and you still have hours on your brace schedule left to go... toss some of your under-brace tanks in the freezer! No need to even soak them in water and make a mess. They'll cool you right down for a little bit!

What about daytime clothes? Check online for bloggers, vloggers, and social media accounts all about brace fashion. There are *tons* of options out there for pieces that will smoothly fit under and over your brace. It may take some time to find such articles that you also *like*, but those online warriors can give you ideas about where to start. Baggy sweaters are the easiest and coziest go-to (even without a brace), but skirts, jeans, and cute tops can still be on the table. It might take a while to engineer those outfits with the brace, but give it time. Try one size larger than usual to fit over the brace.

No matter what, it's about wearing what makes you feel good. Some of us prefer trying on clothes in-store rather than ordering online. That way we can see how the article falls on us right away and make a decision about its comfort within five seconds. Your friends and family would probably love a little fashion adventure at the mall to help *you* – the model – design a new wardrobe. If you're not quite used to wearing the brace yet, go on a shopping spree without it, or order some new items online that *can be returned*.

As you get used to your brace, you'll also learn just how tight it should be. The orthotist usually marks it on the Velcro straps when they're on the front, but it can be harder to gauge when they're on the back. Careful not to tighten it *extra* tight with the incorrect goal of "the tighter it is, the better it will work." Tighter brace does not equal quicker results. Tighten it the way your orthotist teaches you and don't go overboard to the point that you feel like a cartoon being crunched into an old-style corset. By the way, some people who have never seen a back brace before may actually ask you if it's a corset.

What about sports and general activities? Much like anything else, this takes some getting used to. You learn very quickly to bend at the knees instead of at the hips. You'll figure out how to lift things up and find work-arounds for anything too twisty. Depending on your hours, you may be allowed to take your brace off for specific activities and sports. For example, if you are a singer and attend choir practice, your brace is probably affecting your diaphragm breathing and power to sing – see if you can exchange your brace hours to have choir practice brace-free. Or maybe you already have permission to have brace-free soccer practice. Just be sure to put your brace somewhere safe and out of harm's way – you don't want any soccer balls hitting this expensive custom piece of equipment!

The back brace has been a scoliosis tool for a *long time*. How many people must have had back braces of all kinds through the years? Consider the great-grandmas who had old-school back braces that were casts made out of plaster.[26] Ours are feathers compared to theirs *and* we can take them off easily! People from all generations are almost always ready to talk about back braces and tips, online or in-person. Set out to find such a community where the common ground is littered in retired and active braces.

Some people's closest friendships have been created over back braces. Maybe you'll find yourself traveling somewhere new to meet a friend or attend a conference with bracers from all over the world. When flying, security will likely be curious about your brace and pat you down. Once you've hung it around your roller bag to get to your gate (if your hours permit you to do so), ask the flight crew to store your brace safely in an overhead compartment – those seats are uncomfortable and restrictive even *without* a brace.

You're not alone going into this. You won't be the first, and you won't be the last. Talk to others with braces – you might just learn something new!

Staying warm during cold months

Bracers tend to have no issue *whatsoever* with those cold winter days and nights, as their cocoons keep them warm. Cool days allow for big, soft, cozy sweaters and layered styles. Cool nights offer the perfect balance between retaining body heat and not overheating. Hunker down and enjoy that weather!

The nighttime "shell waddle"

Have you ever put on your night brace, gone to sleep, and then woken up with some natural biological urge that requires walking?

As it was explained to me, night braces are bent at more aggressive angles than day braces and need fuller coverage to do their job since they have fewer hours to be effective. My Charleston bending brace did not leave much room for graceful movement. If for some reason I needed to get up in the middle of the night for a snack, I had a brilliant plan in place – brilliant, but also comedic.

Rather than rip the brace open, awakening my entire family with the sound of three giant Velcro straps, I tried to keep my brace on and get out of bed. I would creep my feet and legs across the surface of my mattress until they hung over the edge and then use my arms to push myself up and off in one quick sweep. My feet would hit the floor almost at the same time my torso came off the mattress. After this all-in-one test of biceps and balance, my hips would be structurally locked into place so my legs needed to pick up the slack and get me to the desired location. The only option? Hop from one foot to the other, penguin-style! It became known in our household as the "shell waddle."

Thankfully I knew the layout of my house very well and could navigate it in the dark, knowing where to turn, where to look out for obstacles on the floor, and approximately how many waddle-hops it took from the bed to the midnight snack. It was like my own house was the "neutral zone" in a video game, where I couldn't fall off any cliffs or run into any baddies. Worst thing that could happen was a little stumble into a door frame, which I always laughed off thinking, "That probably hurt the door more than it hurt me and my shell." Hotels and friends' houses were another story. They were a jump right up to the boss level of the video game. I'd have no idea of the floor plan, no clue of obstacles on the floor or fragile lamps – just a Hail Mary hop around the place until I got to where I needed to be.

Thinking back, there were a great many "boss levels" with that brace. After a while, I instituted a couple of rules: Snack before bed to escape the need to waddle, and don't drink anything past 8:00 p.m. to prevent the midnight-Velcro-wake-up-call for my family. Rest assured you can beat every single one of these brace challenges because *spoiler alert* *you* are the real boss. Get creative and *womp* all these brace complexities. Leave them in the dust and move on to taking care of yourself.

A final piece of advice: *Stay away from the stairs with a night brace.* If you absolutely have to use the stairs, rip open your brace and ditch it before venturing onto any steep incline or decline. Nobody wants a brace shell *and* a cast shell at the same time. Take it easy on yourself and take care of *you*. Remember that you're temporarily wearing it to take care of your health in the best way possible. This is a unique opportunity we have as teenagers to use our remaining growth to stop scoliosis from progressing. Thank you, brace, for being there and working hard.

Scoliosis at school

To hide scoliosis or not to hide scoliosis? That may be a question.

Sure, you could hide it physically with clothes, but what about hiding the simple fact that you *have* AIS – not telling anybody anything about it, not giving a glimmer of information about your health, not providing any explanation for your medical appointments or emotions... full incognito scoliosis! If you're thinking about handling this weird sliver of your life by hiding away like too many of us used to do, I totally get where you're coming from. But how much energy is wasted to hide it? Energy you could be using instead to make friends, create memories, and have fun.

The resounding advice from *all* warriors who went through high school with scoliosis or a brace: Don't hide it.

You're going through *way* more than you should have to deal with right now, and going through it alone is unnecessarily tougher. Most warriors who have become adults – "warrior elders" – or are scoli-support group leaders will tell you that scoliosis and braces are *nothing* to be ashamed of, that it *does not* change who you are as a person, and that it *does not* define you. Those adults who look back on their concealed time, and the tons of energy spent hiding and worrying about it, now wish they'd been much more open about it.

School is still a time to make friends and have fun! A brace or scoliosis should not limit any of that. But it can be hard to strut around confidently, paying no mind to people laughing *around* you in the halls (the odds that they're laughing *at* you are very, very, very small, by the way). So make *every thing* your friend – your brace and your back – and make some friends along the way. Even just telling a couple of friends or teachers at school can get rid of a *ton* of stress; you don't need to single-handedly deal with scoliosis from 8:00 a.m. to 3:00 p.m. every weekday. Being open with the people you feel comfortable with can strengthen those friendships further, and the better the friendships you have, the more confident you feel! Scoliosis doesn't want to make you completely alone; it just wants to make you a little twisted.

The majority of high schoolers worry about what other people think of them on a good day, never mind when you have a bonus medical condition. *Especially* when it's something most people know nothing about! Not to make it seem that one ailment is worse than another – they're all a pain – but something like diabetes or chickenpox is well known and understood by most. Not so much for scoliosis. If you mention it, you may get blank stares or maybe even some questions. Talking about scoliosis can feel weird at the start, but it gets easier the more you do it. You may not be ready or want to explain scoliosis to every single person. Guess what? It's not your job to educate the masses. It's just your job to take care of yourself and ensure you have a good support system in place to talk with, like your family and a couple of best friends.

I only told a handful of my closest school friends about my scoliosis in my senior year once surgery was needed. They didn't know I'd been wearing a brace or was in constant pain at all. And guess what? They were *immensely* supportive! Most knew little to nothing about scoliosis, but they asked questions about what it was, what it was doing to me, and how they could help. One knew all about it already because her mother had scoliosis and surgery – what are the odds! Scoliosis may not be extremely common, but it is certainly not that rare.

So how can we make those first few days at school in a brace go nice and smooth? First of all, talk to your school's administration. Ask to go to school after hours one day, once the halls are empty, to test drive your new brace. If you were assigned a bottom-level locker, ask to switch to a top-level one that is easier to access without bending. Figure out how to fit it in your locker, how to sit in classroom chairs (sometimes edges can catch), and generally how to move around with it outside of home. A trial run can ease some first-day worries!

If you're still figuring out how to put it on and take it off quickly, see if there is a room you can use to do that in peace and quiet, grabbing a little stretch at the same time. Ask to leave a pillow in class to make sitting comfier, and request a second set of textbooks to leave at home to make your backpack lighter. You may also want to let them know that you need longer bathroom breaks – especially at the beginning.

A final note on hiding "it": High school is a super weird time that comes with the unique social pressures and complexities of being a teenager. If you're there now, know that it gets better. *Way* better. Hang in there and keep talking about your experience with people close to you

Joking with your friends

Some scolis and bracers need time and self-education before they're ready to open up and talk to other people about their scoliosis. It can take some strength and courage. Don't rush it if you're not ready.

Lots of people try to hide their orthodontic braces when they first get them too. But, much like scoliosis braces, it's so much easier to smile through that phase rather than hide away and not speak to anybody. Telling a couple of friends and using laughter as medicine can be fun!

It took me a bit to get used to my own night brace. Once I got comfortable enough and told my best friend about it, sleepovers started back up again! Those were the only opportunities she had to see the brace and, bless her inquisitive mind, ask me questions about it. She really wanted to understand what was happening and cared enough to help any way she could.

In usual sleepover shenanigans, at some point a pillow is thrown and some kind of scuffle breaks out. What a perfect opportunity to lean in to the humor that you're wearing your own personal exoskeleton! That's right, toss a pillow my way. Watch as I laugh it off and throttle you right back. No pillow can make it through my rock-hard "abs"! Going to try to tickle me instead? Good luck! You can't get to half of me, but I sure can tickle *you*. I win!

Some friends, who know that tickling through a brace is impossible, poke and surprise the bracer through the brace holes. Some bracers let their friends endearingly "knock" on their brace when they want to chat, much like knocking on a door. Some bracers have fun watching boys in class freak out when they knock on their much stronger plastic "abs." A habit of drumming fingers against it often forms – a much better habit than biting your nails!

As annoying as braces and scoliosis can be, it truly teaches you to look differently at life's little moments. Don't take life too seriously! Find the lightness and humor in your brace and, as an extension, in life.

LESSONS AND REMINDERS

Breathing

Sometimes scoliosis can affect the cardiovascular system, which includes the heart and lungs. There are numerous biomechanical calculations for how scoliosis can structurally affect the amount of air we can take in – which we are not going to dive into here.[27] What you are likely to notice in your own scoliosis, though, is how the thoracic curve can restrict lung expansion on one side. But that's not the only thing at play here. Some bracers wear a tight brace for years, preventing the belly and diaphragm from fully expanding all day long and using the chest and shoulders to move air instead.

We don't always consider "the breath" as teenagers – especially if we're not athletes, actors, or musicians, where breathing is key to performance. Breathing is just something the body does naturally because it's key to life, after all! But the breath can also play a key part in managing and countering scoliosis.[28] New brace designs are even considering the power of breath now.

Don't worry, different ways of breathing can be learned. A large part of scoli-yoga and PSSE corrective exercises is all about how to use the breath. Their professionals know how to get you started – how to breathe *into* the concavities, how to use the diaphragm to breathe, how to breathe deep and slow... It's another piece of the body puzzle you can learn about. Just like any other corrective exercises your expert asks you to do, learning to breathe a different way can take time, practice, and patience. Nothing happens overnight! It takes time to convince your muscles and your brain to work a different way, get used to the feeling, and stick with it.

It's also worth mentioning that a study in 2016 gathered data showing a potential link between patients with scoliosis and heart abnormalities. This study went on to recommend echocardiography testing for scoliosis patients so that any potential heart problem could be caught sooner rather than later.[29]

Knowledge of your body

When I was in high school, our biology class ran out of time for teaching the last part of the curriculum, which happened to be "The Human Body." You'd think that would be important enough to cover at the beginning of the semester... but I digress. We never went back to cover those chapters, and it was never discussed again. By some coincidence, that was around the same time I received my diagnosis. Little did I know that my real education was about to begin.

You may be new to this club and completely overwhelmed with all of the medical mumbo-jumbo and vertebrae diagrams that are constantly being floated by you. Worry not! *Of course* this seems overwhelming to you: It's all brand-new information, and a lot of it at that! Give it time. You will slowly begin to understand how the vertebrae, discs, and muscles in your back work;

why things hurt; and how you can work with it all to improve your situation. The body is a wonderful machine and you are a junior mechanic. In no time, you'll become an expert yourself.

Instead of a fine public school education on this topic, I was schooled by doctors and therapists. I learned how the components of our bodies can work with or against each other, and by extension how best to alleviate resulting pain for *my body*. I began to gather information about the impacts of scoliosis on the body, and I continue to learn about these topics.

To be clear, should you go through with surgery, your post-op education about the human body (in particular *your* body) shouldn't stop. You should continue learning how to live in this muscle meat sack: how to stretch, workout, and care for it. Maybe you already have a scoli-pro teaching you. Maybe you're working your way through different treatment types, retaining what works for you. Maybe you've been gathering up exercises over the years. You're becoming your own expert in taking care of *you*.

Now, would I have rather had "The Human Body" education that the high school curriculum promised me instead of scoliosis? Yes, of course. But just like every other high school subject, I would have purged everything from that musty old textbook from my mind the second the final exam was over. I would not have been in as good a position to support my health in the long run. This diagnosis is a "hands on" bonus education from Professor Scoliosis that will stick with you forever if you seek out good information.

It's not life-threatening

This ailment is a pain in the butt. It sucks. When I ask warriors what emotion comes to mind when they think of scoliosis, a common answer is "frustration." However, most scoliosis on its own is not life-threatening.

Every experience you go through with your back will teach you something about life or about yourself. You may have days where you're waiting with bated breath to see if it will hurt, but you don't have to worry about it terminating you. You just have to live with it by your side – probably more on one side than the other. (Scoliosis humor!)

You are not alone

It may seem like it at times, especially if you've never met another scoli in real life, but *you are not alone*. You're not alone having scoliosis. You're not alone wearing a brace. You're not alone considering spinal surgery. Maybe down the line you'll also need to remind yourself you're not the only one with a spinal fusion.

Many warriors feel like they're the only one on the planet with this *thing*, and that nobody else understands them. Sometimes this lasts until they speak to another scoli online or meet one in real life and see their brace or scar.

Things used to be very different. Even a decade ago, there was next to no information readily available about how to live with scoliosis or what it meant for a person's future. The only scoliosis resources available were complicated medical articles filled with scary pictures and negative forums about pain and low body confidence. The articles were often about outdated procedures and rare surgery mistakes. The internet at your fingertips, yet nothing of actual use. Even locating somebody else close to your age who could relate and say, "I know just what you're talking about!" was tricky.

But those days are long gone now! The internet is jam-packed with blogs, podcasts, videos, and e-books ready to answer as many questions as possible. The online scoliosis community has grown to include support groups all over the world. Look for some in your region, get involved, and seek out similar people. It may feel out of your comfort zone, but remember that everybody in these groups has a shared experience through their spines – you'll be surprised at how many people say, "Oh my gosh I thought that only happened with *my* back!"

One-on-one more your style? There are fantastic opportunities for scoli elders to answer questions about bracing or surgery if you're just beginning the process. (I've listed them in the "Resources" section at the end of the book.) You can take part either as a patient or volunteer... maybe eventually moving *from* patient *to* volunteer!

Take the support, find common ground in the scoliosis lifestyle, and encourage each other. So many of us who wish these resources and networks had been set up years ago are finally connecting online now and saying, "I wish I knew there were others out there who spoke my language and knew exactly what it all felt like." Don't go through this alone. This should not be isolating, even though it certainly can feel that way at times.

The Scoliosis Journey for Surgery

There are often so many fears and unknowns when it comes to a surgery – in our case, a spinal fusion for scoliosis – that it can be tough to compile all the questions you want answers to. In this section, we'll go over what to expect during your hospital stay, how to prepare for surgery and recovery, and what your return home may look like. Patients of vertebral body tethering (VBT) – a surgical procedure for scolis who still have a lot of growing to do that implants a flexible cord placed under tension on either side the spine[30] – will find in this section many tips and guidance shared between both fusion and VBT surgeries. My experience, however, is with fusion surgery, so it will be the focus.

Here is what real life preparing and recovering from spinal fusion scoliosis surgery can look and feel like.

HOSPITAL TIME

Setting the surgery date

Gone are the woes of the brace. The decision of "do we operate or do we wait?" has been finalized. You've done your research on surgery methods, hospitals, and surgeons – yes, you *can* get second, third, or even fourth opinions from different surgeons. (See the "Resources" section for interviews with surgeons.) You were honest with your surgeon about how you're feeling, what you want to be able to do after surgery (do you do any specific sports?), and your recovery timeline – it's important to be honest with your surgeon. You and your surgeon will have discussed the goals and plan, and the date has been booked.

Knowing the date can bring immense relief. If it's all you can think about, that's totally normal. You may even write it in your calendar or have a countdown on the go!

You may want it to arrive so you can get it over with, remove some pain, and move on with your life. You also may be hesitant to hit that little box on your calendar because you don't know what your life beyond it will look like. You can think about all the prep, all the risks, all the odds, all the pain relief, all the possibilities of what your life post-surgery may hold. It is a huge help to some warriors to journal their feelings leading up to a surgery. There are so many appointments, questions, and mysteries of the future. It's calming to get your thoughts out on paper, and then it's fascinating to re-read them years later to see who you were at that moment and who you've grown into.

As exciting as that upcoming event may be, don't forget to keep making memories and having fun! Pause any thoughts about things you *can't* control by doing things you *can* control. Make sure to remain active (or get active if you're not already), and continue making healthy nutrition choices. Find some time for fun with people whose company you enjoy or sports you won't be able to do for a few months during recovery. Some warriors make a pre-fusion list of such activities and set out to cross them all off: roller skating, skiing, snowboarding, golfing, jumping on a trampoline, going to a rage room, axe-throwing, hiking, horseback riding... Your friends may also have some fun ideas to contribute. Just take care during all of these activities not to injure yourself – you're supposed to be taking the best care possible of yourself, remember!

Once again, to each their own. You do *you*! Everybody is wired differently, and we all have a unique perspective of the world around us. Likely how we approach surgery is influenced by our past and the people closest to us.

Hospital prep

We'll get into surgery details later, but for now, let's chat "setup." You may be surprised at how many things you can prepare for ahead of time to make your surgery recovery that much smoother. Here are some things to consider, generously shared by fusioneers around the planet.

First of all, what should you bring? The usual medical paperwork, hairbrush, and toothbrush, of course. How about some comfy socks, a teddy bear, a preferred body pillow, phone/tablet and charger, lip balm and moisturizer, dry shampoo, and face wipes? You may want to include a silk pillowcase to make sliding pillows under your head easier, since lifting yourself up is hard to do at first. Don't worry about brain-exercising activities, like books or knitting – you're there to recover. Your brain doesn't need even more exercising during that phase. A book of word searches is about as much work as you'll want to put in. iPads or phones loaded with games can be fun, but be aware that looking down for a long time may strain your neck and thoracic zones.

You'll be in hospital gowns most of the time, so it's always a comfort to have an article of clothing or soft blanket from home. Button-down pajamas are great, since raising your arms will be tough for a few days. The simpler it is to put on the article of clothing, the better! As far as footwear, you can bring socks with no-slip sticky pads under them or shoes with no lacing required. Sandals with elastics all around, for example, but not flip-flops as they're a tripping hazard. Don't forget to bring very loose clothes for when you finally get to go home!

Let's get some potential "surprises" out of the way. You may lose some weight post-op. You're not exercising or moving much, and many patients have trouble keeping food down. Some people are allergic to anesthesia, which causes vomiting and makes it harder to gain weight. Getting in shape and eating well (bulking up, or as some people call it, "pre-hab") before surgery helps put both your mind and body in the best state possible. After surgery, you're unlikely to have a huge appetite, so eating small snacks throughout the day will help with gaining back the weight.

There will be a few people taking care of you in the hospital. Ask your caregiver to bring a pen and paper to log each type and time of medication given to you, just to make sure you're getting all you need. Everybody there is hardworking and well-meaning, but sometimes things can be missed (just like any job). If something doesn't seem right, you or your caregiver need to speak up.

On a related topic, work out your drug plan for when you are discharged from the hospital *before* you go in for surgery. This very much depends on your hospital, country, and doctor situation, but you want to make sure your medication plan is concrete. Find out how much the hospital will be giving you (how many days' worth), and make sure you have access to your family doctor immediately afterwards to get more prescription medication if needed. (It's not like you can walk into any clinic and demand opioids.) Maybe you already have a direct line to your doctor or appointments booked in advance. Excellent! The recommendation here is to know what the next couple of weeks post-surgery are going to look like, instead of trying to track down doctors and drugs at the last minute.

Ask your care team beforehand about any other preparations you can take to make your recovery as smooth as possible while in hospital. Ask the weird questions and talk to other fusioneers – they may give you additional tips and heads-ups!

> **Dear Parents:** Don't forget about yourselves through all of this. Bring something to keep you busy and comfy during the surgery hours. A book, a coloring book, some music, a cozy blanket... you will be spending quite some time at the hospital during surgery and recovery alongside your patient!

Operation day

Well, here we are. Looks like the best course of action is some surgery. Worry not, we have a plan for that!

Let's flit through the appointments running up to the surgery – there will be a few. You may have a couple of extra ones for blood work, depending on your iron levels and blood transfusion plans (yours, family members, or blood bank).

Your caregivers will be given instructions on when to arrive, how to prep, and when to stop feeding you the night before. (That's how all operations operate.) If any paperwork is given to you well in advance of the surgery day, hold on to it and review it closer to the day – there are a lot of emotions at play, and you may not retain all the information right away. Let's zero in on the hospital experience itself.

Below is a general overview based on articles, personal interviews, and personal experience. Every country and hospital is different, so don't be shy about asking for the day's agenda in advance. Some hospitals offer pre-op teaching sessions and walk-throughs of the surgery rooms, going over the team members and the hardware that will be used. This can address many questions and unknowns.

Early on surgery day, you first meet with a little squad of people in an office you've never been in before and will never be in again. There is a review of the procedure to be taken, which vertebrae will be fused, who the team will be, and how long it will take. It is recommended that you braid your hair (if it's long enough) into two crisp, tight braids. This style will keep it out of your way, and seems to be the favorite patient hairstyle for the entire hospital stay!

During the first couple of checkpoints, you will receive your fancy plastic hospital bracelet and change into a hospital gown (just one). A nurse will also plaster some numbing cream on you to prepare for the IV lines. (Mine were on the back of both my hands.)

That part will zip by, and next thing you know you'll be in the pre-op holding room (the waiting room before the operating room). You will probably be allowed to hang on to a teddy bear for comfort, and a parent will be permitted to accompany you. There is no shame in holding a teddy bear or a parent's hand at any point throughout this day, by the way. The build-up of getting to the operation may peak by this point, and the minutes may seem to stretch. Many of us recall an eerie mix of calm and anticipation washing over us in that weird in-between space. If you're not feeling calm, you can ask for something to help calm you down – the hospital team is there to help you out.

Finally, you are wheeled into the last room of the "operation" portion: the operating room (OR). If your parent is accompanying you, they will be dressed in protective hospital garb complete with booties and mask. Your teddy bear can cruise in with you too! This is a real operation room complete with lights, machines, surgical tools (either covered with a surgical drape or uncovered), and a whole team waiting to take the very best care of you: surgeons, nurses, assistants, orderlies, anesthesiologists. Some patients love it; others don't. (That's why we're not all doctors!) It's okay if you don't like it – don't be shy about telling a nurse beforehand or asking for help. Some sedation may begin before you're brought into the OR, or the anesthesia process will begin immediately once inside, sending you off into a deep sleep.

Next thing you know, you'll wake up in the intensive care unit (ICU) recovery room! This is intense care (aptly named) that you need for the first day or so post-op. Your care here will be the absolute best you will ever experience in your life. You will have a few temporary pieces of equipment helping you out, like an oxygen mask or feeding tube and a catheter. Whatever else is hooked up to you is for your own health and safety – no need to know it all. Your parents finally get to come see you, but waking from anesthesia makes you groggy and disoriented (or as my father said, "Drugged like a horse"). You'll have a *lot* of painkillers on the go here while vacationing in the world's comfiest, cushiest ICU bed.

My only memory – and it's the foggiest one of my whole life – was *desperately* trying to text my friends that I was through surgery... on a *flip phone*. (Millennials, you know what I'm talking about – that's a challenge on a sober day, never mind on a high-as-a-kite hospital day. Generation Z, you have no clue what cell phone life used to be like – get outta here with your touch screen voice-clip messaging.) My nurse was a tough, peppy young lady who took wonderful care of me and joked with me in my quest to text my friends. She even came to check on me in my post-ICU room to see how I was doing, where she told me I had barely been able to get one letter punched out in my phone in ICU before dropping back into a sedated state. Apparently I entertained her as she worked one of the world's toughest professions: nursing.

Surgery séjour

Everything is good, any complications have been addressed, your feeding tube is gone... time to make some space in the ICU and move to a regular hospital room! If this includes changing beds, how does one move from a plush ICU bed to a regular hospital bed? It's not like you can get up and saunter from one to the other yet. It goes like this: A small team may half roll, half pull you off the ICU bed onto a wooden bridge and then tip you onto your next bed. I doubt there is actually a more graceful way of doing that transfer, but it can feel like you're a ball of raw dough being moved from one counter to another.

That was also the day I learned I would *not* get to choose my own hospital bed – the universe was not with me on that front. I was given what I maintain was the oldest bed somehow still in service at that hospital. While my short roommate had a long, plush bed reminiscent of the ICU with electric adjustment buttons, lights, and tons of padding, I had a wood-and-metal framed bed that was barely my length with what I believe was an old military-issue camping mattress. The kicker was the manual crank at the foot of the bed, which someone *else* had to operate to tilt the back rest up and down. Discuss this with your team *beforehand* so as to avoid my bed situation. Request a bed from this century, since you will want to be in control of adjusting the back of the bed regularly. I cannot emphasize enough how much you will *not* want to feel the vibrations of a manual crank – you will be quite sensitive to all movements at first. Your care team will of course be around to help you re-adjust in bed, propping pillows all around. You may find yourself wanting to sleep a little bit more upright to breathe better and sleep deeper.

Post-op pain is different for everyone. There will be pain initially since your body just went through *a lot* – it has many adjustments and much healing to do! Your first few days out of the ICU and into the recovery phase are going to hurt the most, but that level is completely individual. The excellent news is you are entrusted with a button that controls an IV to self-dose painkillers when it starts feeling very *ow*-y. I am certainly not a big painkiller person, but there are no points for enduring extra pain the first few days. Take a smidge of help! Know that once your time with this button is up, you will still take oral painkillers. The one annoying thing is that you have to wake up every few hours to take your doses, which can kind of get in the way of your deep recovery sleep time (a necessary nuisance, but not a big deal).

Some people need more painkillers to help them out than others. There's no guesstimating this beforehand; just take it one moment at a time and be sure to speak up if you need some medicinal assistance for the pain. Nobody wants to *over*drug or *under*drug you, but also nobody knows how you're feeling. The pain should not be *so bad* that you can't function. Your parents/caregivers should also be your advocates and be able to say, "This isn't enough; we aren't handling this well." Then again, you may be just fine with the dosage they set you up with initially.

Girls, FYI: You are likely to get your period while recovering in your hospital room. Don't worry if you wake up to blood on your bedsheets – it may not be from your back. As it was explained to us: your body knows something big is happening and it doesn't want any chance of you getting pregnant – that would simply be too much for it to handle. Even if you never had your period before, it may begin that week. Don't worry about it, though; the angelic nurses have pads at the ready. Honestly, you'll be on so many painkillers, you won't care at all.

What about food? You'll be on a liquid diet for the first little bit and may not hold down food too well. You may very well cry when you're handed your first piece of bread. That's okay! Bodies can't handle too much serious food after such an experience. The nurses will bring you snacks and instruct your parents which foods should absolutely be avoided. Know that *any red food* is banned. Your well-meaning mother should absolutely *not* bring in homemade red Jell-O because you're sick and tired of the hospital's lemon Jell-O. She will get in trouble for that. (Sorry, Mom.) The hospital needs to know if that's blood in your vomit... or just Jell-O.

My mom, bless her heart, made soup from scratch at home, brought it to the hospital, got somebody to help sit me up in a chair-like contraption, and convinced me to eat a whole bowl of wholesome nutrients after a few days... which I promptly threw up. (Again, sorry, Mom!) Towards the end of my stay, I was ready for my best friend to visit. We chatted, laughed, and shared the teeniest snack-sized bag of gummy treats. This was promptly followed by the now-immortal line of our friendship paired with a panicked look: "Get me something to throw up in." It wasn't a question but, rather, a statement with a very short timeline. She grabbed some tiny metal bowl, held it out to me, and within seconds her thumb was dipping into a warm container with floating gummies. Now, if that isn't friendship, I don't know what is. All this to say: There's no shame in throwing up post-op; it happens to many of us.

Rest, painkillers, and food are all super important, but equally important is getting up and walking. The sooner you get up and take those first steps, the stronger your chances of swift recovery and the sooner you go home. Every fusioneer is different, but it helps to psych yourself up mentally about this and take a dose of painkiller *beforehand* – time your walks with your pain meds. The hospital's physical therapists are going to swing by and encourage you to walk. If you really aren't up for it at that moment, say, "Yes, I will go for a walk, but could you please come back in half an hour once I've had my pain meds?"

This comes down to determination. It's not going to be super fun or easy on day one, but don't shy away from it. Find that inner power to stand up and take a step – even if it's *one* step that's the longest, slowest step ever. Hey, you did it, great job! Next thing you know, you'll be taking slow walks around the hallway, holding on to the railing, or wearing out a circle in the floor of your room.

Sitting is another new activity the physical therapists have you try out. It's the same deal here: allow pain medication to help, mentally know this is important to your recovery, and take it a few minutes at a time. Heads up that the sitting may be more uncomfortable than the walking.

Bodies are strong and heal remarkably well. (We were *all* amazed at how quickly recovery happens!) The first few days are the most challenging, but each day gets a bit easier. Take the time to rest, but *do not give up*! Recovery is *not* linear – there will be ups and downs.

Family support is the #1 super tool for your scoli toolkit. *Let* your family support you. They love you! And don't kid yourself... this is about as tough on them as it is on you. Parents are encouraged to stay at the hospital during the day and night in the fold-out chair/bed combo ever-present in patient rooms. Most of these hospital stays are just a few days; you may be home in under a week. You can also keep all of the loving "get well soon" cards near your bed and read them (or ask somebody to read them to you).

All fusioneers have praised their care teams who addressed their fears and questions. Even those patients who had complications and required additional care were grateful for their teams and wholly respected that they treated them so lovingly. Remember that every single fusioneer has a different experience. There are tons of firsthand blogs and social media accounts on this topic – I strongly encourage you to look up other surgical and recovery sagas.

Side-effects may include...

Nobody likes thinking about this topic, but the reality of it is that sometimes "extra" things happen. There are risks that come with every surgery out there. Always. But those risks usually have extremely minuscule odds of actually happening and large odds of *not* happening. There's also a risk that you could walk outside right now and be run over by a truck. Let's leave the deep discussion of risks between you and your surgeon. Most of this should be covered in your pre-op meeting.

A couple of worries that have come up in numerous conversations do bear mentioning here: infection and nerve damage. That's because this surgery is quite invasive and takes quite a few hours.[31] If you are worrying about either, know that we *all* had a smidge of worry about them. Some ladies who never voiced their worries pre-op asked if their legs were working mere moments after shrugging off the anesthetic. Some had worries about infection and never had any. Others were not too worried about either and did experience one. There's no planning for it. Keep an eye out for signs of infection especially once you are discharged from the hospital.

It may be interesting to know that during surgery they use a breathing tube to monitor your breathing while you're on your stomach. These tubes cause a certain level of hoarseness for everybody and in odd cases are so irritating that the voice is lost. Since air supply is so crucial to the operation, the anesthetic team monitors this very closely. Feeding tubes are also in play during the hospital stay, the most common being a nasogastric tube, which goes in through the nose, down the esophagus, and into the stomach for additional nutritional intake.

Sometimes bodies don't want to go back to their regularly scheduled programs right away. Additional blood transfusions may be needed while recovering in the care of the hospital. Catheters may need to go home with the patient for a few days. Every body is very different, and the trained team of specialists will be watching out for you, tending to all of these cares. If you don't know what's going on or something really doesn't feel right, ask or have your caregiver speak up for you!

You cannot choose your own adventure in what will happen or not happen. But you *can* do your research to select your doctor, hospital, and anesthesiologist so you can feel the most at ease with and confident about this process as possible.

What about long-term post-op? Well, that's also one great big unknown! Some people experience varied pains. Others have fractures. Sometimes metalwork comes loose. Others are A-okay. With the immobility of the fusion location, surrounding areas can get tight since you can't really move them around to stretch. (Exercise balls and massages come in very handy!) A large factor of your long-term post-op health is what we keep circling back to: *taking care of your own overall health!*

Your new side-effect could be summed up as ongoing care and education. Diet, exercise, mental health, social support, learning about your unique body and back! Just because a bracing or surgery is over, it doesn't mean the scoliosis is all gone and we can neglect our bodies. No way! The more you learn, the better you can take care of yourself.

Pills and needles

Have trouble swallowing pills? Oh, you'll figure out some way to get it done while in the hospital. You will have IV medicine for the first little bit, but it's not advisable to stay on heavy opioid painkillers for too long, so pills will replace that rather quickly. And trust me, you're going to *want* to gobble them up when they're delivered to your room in that majestic paper cup.

I was *terrible* at swallowing pills pre-op. I used to chew my over-the-counter painkillers in high school to get them down. (Don't do that.) That could no longer happen with hospital-grade painkillers (and whatever else they were feeding me in pill form). So I devised a way to trick my tongue from grabbing the pills mid-swallow. Take a little bite of food – any food – and stash the pill inside it. Then swallow in one big Trojan-horse pill gulp.

Scared of needles too? You may not be as scared after your hospital stay! (That fear went right out of my mind once I was so immersed in it.) Those needles are caring for you and feeding you all of the necessary fluids and medicines, after all. You may still not *like* getting shots or seeing blood drawn, but if you have a wild fear about it before, it may be dampened. The hospital stay may surprise you with little life skills.

Sneezing

That force that comes from deep within courtesy of allergies, a cool breeze, or just the whimsy of life. That force that builds up to rattle your ribs, painfully unearth every knot under your shoulder blades, engage your muscular imbalances, and throw your neck backwards. Too bad it can't frighten your spine into alignment... if only.

It kind of makes sense that sneezing can hurt when you learn that the majority of your body is involved in a sneeze. All hands on deck to get whatever is tickling your nose out of there – your throat, your chest, your diaphragm, a bit of an ab workout... all parts of your anatomy that encircle your spine.[32]

One piece of advice is to sit down as soon as a sneeze begins to build – giving it only the upper body to jostle – while absorbing most of the shock through the stabilized seat.

That's all manageable out of a brace and well after recovery... But what about during recovery immediately after surgery? If a sneeze must happen, it can be quite painful. Your brain is not going to change how it sneezes just for you, so all of those body parts are still going to contract. That's not the most pleasant sensation when your body is adjusting to so many changes! You can't run to a chair to absorb any impact, but you can grab a bunch of pillows from your stash and hold them against your chest. The same goes for coughing.

On a related note: Throwing up in a recovery state is also unpleasant, aside from the regular reasons. Many muscles also contract for this reaction, and your body naturally leans forward as it happens. You may not have leaned forward yet post-op so this can be a new and jarring sensation. Once again, the nurses are there to help you, hold your hair, and supply painkillers as needed. It's brief, and you will make it through – we all did!

Scars

What surgery would be complete without a nice new scar? The ultimate battle wound. Proof that you went through something extreme, and that you are fantastically strong. A vision of a pirate grimacing with a worldly twinkle in their eyes comes to mind.

We have some options here for surgical scars. There's the *Thoracic Treat*, hanging out at/above the bra line and peeking out above the back of low-cut clothes. The *Lumbar Looker*, dancing along the lower back and popping out below crop-tops. Of course, the *Double Down*, handling both thoracic and lumbar curves doing double duty in one long, thin white line. If you're going with some of the new "fusionless" surgery options out there, your scar may be on the side instead – a shiny new *Sideways Slit*.

But wait, there's more! Depending on the needs of your surgery, you may have had a scar on your hip or rib. What about the leftover scars from where drain bags and IVs were plugged in? There are many little reminders of *strength*.

If you don't love your scar right off the bat, please be as gentle with yourself as you can. The back scar really lightens up over time, going from purple-red to faint white. Remember, scars tell a tale and are a reminder that you lived through something powerful. You are so strong, and you have the badge of strength to prove it (not that you ever need to). They may be tender, tingly, or numb for a bit, but nobody sees them as much as you do. If you don't love 'em quite yet, still keep on moisturizing, sunscreening, and caring for them. If something about the scarring really bothers you as time goes by, there is always the potential for some plastic surgery.

Despite the inevitability of scars, this is a perfect opportunity to take a pause and think about how this surgery *used to be* in the olden days. Lots of new surgical methods are being developed and enhanced! The lookbook for scars will continue to expand, but the scars themselves are likely to get smaller and smaller. Medicine is – and continues to get – better!

Less curve, less prominence, less pain, more height

This may just be one small entry here, but it holds an immense amount of weight as this is the ultimate point of fusion surgery.

While it doesn't "cure" scoliosis, fusion surgery can prevent moderate-to-severe curves from increasing over time. Unfortunately, there exists no magic crystal ball that can say how much more each curve would progress over the years *without* surgery. Many of us had surgery not so much for the cosmetic aspect, but to reduce pain and prevent the curves from growing. Any surgery can be scary, and while not everybody reaps the full potential rewards, many fusioneers say this one changed their life for the better.

The cosmetic aspect does also factor in for many surgical decisions. Not only will straightening the spine make you taller, but you're likely to find a self-esteem boost as well. Prominences that may have bothered you before *may* be reduced. You may even find it easier to breathe! Your body may need a couple of weeks to settle into its new form, so do not despair if you don't see it right away. Similarly, if you've been in your scoli-shape for many years, your muscles may need some time to adjust and "let go" of their holding patterns. A massage – once you've been okay-ed by your doctor – a few weeks post-op can help with that; just ask them not to touch the incision if you don't want them to.

If you've already had surgery and a small piece of your mind sometimes pipes up to say, "Well, maybe I could have improved on my own with exercises. Maybe I didn't need to have the fusion," silence that part of your mind. It's done. You're fused. There's no point spending energy on that "what if." Living in the past gets you nowhere fast. It's time to live in the present… for the future.

HOME TIME

Household prep

Here's a common surgery question: "Is there anything we can get ready ahead of time to make recovery easier?" The short answer: "Yes."

But first, let's plan to get you home in that post-op car ride. You'll want to sit on a pillow or fluffy blanket and stack pillows all around you to isolate yourself from feeling the bumps in the road. (Fair warning that you *will* feel every dent in the road right through your new spine.) Ask your chauffeur to avoid potholes where possible. As you recover, car rides will hurt less and less, but right now you are still very much healing.

Aside from the car, complete as many preparations as you can *before* operation day. Work with your surgeon to understand the recovery timeline and what you should absolutely avoid (bending, lifting, twisting) and continue to do (walking, moisturizing). Also find out where your incision is going to be. You'll still need to make some tweaks to the best-laid plans and get creative, but you can get some options in place.

Raising your arms after having back surgery when your wound is still tender and healing is simply not going to happen. Even lifting your toothbrush may seem like too much at first. It's going to take time before you'll be able to toss on your regular t-shirts. Nor will you be able to smoothly bend forward to put on pants, balancing on one leg at a time to foist your foot through a cloth hole. Solution: Wear underwear and invest in nightgowns, button-ups, or men's extra-large t-shirts! Find some with great big loose sleeves and a wide body that can slide on without raising the arms too much. (Dads, lend us your soft shirts!) You're not out to impress anybody right now. Your sole job is healing, and nobody around you should care what costume you do that in. If you must wear pants, wear loose pants. Fighting and tugging up tight pants is beyond frustrating and totally unnecessary.

Ladies, you will at some point heal up enough to want to put on a bra. But wait... most bras have hooks along the back, right where your healing fusion incision is! Good thing you went out *before* your surgery and bought loose bras that go on like a backpack, with the clasps in the *front*. Something with wide, flat straps around the back and sides, which cause no lumps when leaning against them. Might take some searching, but they are definitely out there. When I found mine, I bought every color they had right on the spot. As mentioned above, don't buy pull-on bras (sports bras, for example) since raising your arms will not be pleasant.

You will still have many medications to take, all of which are important to your recovery. This is not something you want to lose track of or confuse, so keep it tight! Parents usually monitor this since patients are in and out of sleep so much. A simple chart on a piece of paper tracking the time, type of med required, and whether you took them is key! You have *got* to drink a lot of fluids after surgery to keep your body hydrated and flush out the drugs. Our bodies are about 55 to 60 percent water[33] – we have to feed them! Solution when lying down: sippy cups or no-spill water bottles. Solution when sitting: straws. No mess and no excuses!

While you're drinking your fluids, think back to how smart you were to ask friends and family for TV and book recommendations in advance! You will want distractions. As many as possible. Zone out into another world and get addicted to something that can keep you entertained for a good amount of time. Back in my day, friends brought over stacks of DVDs and books to keep me occupied. (A few months later, I got to enjoy those movies for the first time all over again since I had no recollection of watching them during my drugged recovery state.) One little thing to be careful about: comedies. Jokes and light humor are great, but non-stop gut-busting hilarity can really hurt. Think about which muscles engage when you laugh... then add a tender incision on top of that. Surprise *ow*.

Regardless of your type and location of surgery, you are going to want to avoid lying directly on your scar. With a scar on your back, you do not want to find yourself fighting to balance on your sides without any aids while horizontal, so invest in a body or maternity pillow to lean forward onto. The hospital team will teach you how to get up from a horizontal position, but doing it alone is tough as heck for the first little bit – you may require some help at home. But what happens if you drank so much from that sippy cup that you need to pee in the middle of the night? Where are your family nurses to help you out? Asleep, of course. Solution: Everybody keeps their charged cell phones at hand at night. Give them a call when you require assistance to get upright, and then thank them profusely!

It can also be rough to get into a seated position alone, particularly if your toilet is low. If you find yourself struggling to sit down on the throne, acquire a toilet seat riser (or proactively acquire one in advance). They're not just for the elderly – they're a marvel for surgery patients too! While you're at that store, find a handle or walker of some sort to assist in pulling you up for the first couple of weeks. You won't need these forever, and after a while you should challenge yourself to use them less and less. Don't worry about this at the hospital – they have it all set up already.

Aside from the toilet, be prepared to rearrange your living space as required. You will be coming home from the hospital feeling beat-up and drugged, so have something set up to waddle directly over to. My parents had the foresight to move my bed from my room on the second floor to the middle of the living area on the main floor. I hobbled in through the doors after slowly clearing the three outdoor steps and went *right* to leaning on the edge of that bed to catch my breath. The day you leave the hospital can be exciting and exhausting – it's a lot!

Your doctors *don't* want you lying down in bed all of the time after surgery, no matter how comfy it may seem. You need to get upright as often as possible (preferably in motion, walking around your house). You are going to want to rest somewhere other than your bed, and those hard wooden kitchen chairs are *not* going to be comfortable. Solution: Get yourself a fluffy, comfy chair. Borrow one from a friend, buy one, take the zero gravity chair from the patio furniture set, or ask grandma to lend you her electric recliner for a few weeks (these can also be rented). If possible, test these out before surgery to see how easily you can get up and out of it (watch out for different zero gravity chair designs). Pile your temporary throne with pillows left, right, and center to add extra clouds of padding all around; adjust it until your nest is just right. Some comfy blankets, a solid grabber-stick, and a coffee table within easy reach would not be turned away either. This is your TV and nap throne for the next few weeks. Enjoy!

No matter what, be sure to *walk, walk, walk* as often as you can, even if it's just for a few minutes at a time (which it will be, at the start). It's the best thing you can do to help you rapidly gain back strength. Use a timer if you want. Set mini goals for yourself to celebrate personal wins at the end of each day. Go outside if the weather is cooperating – just be wary of additional obstacles in the outside world… your living area is likely much more pristine.

All patients and living quarters are different, but one recommendation is to set up a bed or couch centrally to avoid stairs. Some hospitals mandate conquering stairs before the patient can be cleared for discharge, but not all… Stairs were very tricky for me, apparently because my fusion went so low. It took me quite a few days of strengthening through walking before I could confidently make it up our long flight of stairs on my own. This was a main goal I had in mind to work towards, and boy was it worth it! The first thing I did when I got upstairs? Put on my earrings and gave myself a mini-manicure. That was the first inkling of "feeling like myself" once again!

Next comes the goal of that glorious shower. Your bandage during the first few weeks may be water resistant, but it's not likely waterproof. Initially you'll be limited to bird baths in the sink, dry shampoo, and no-rinse shampoo. Since soaking in a bath or standing under hot running water for a long time are out of the question, be extra sure to scrub well with face cloths or face wipes regularly. (By the way, it's disgustingly amazing how quickly dead skin can pile up if you don't wash.)

The days of dry shampoo need to end. But how? My mother and I cried with laughter as we tried to engineer some setup that would get my head under the shower faucet while keeping my back flat and dry. Try and picture the final product: a shower seat on the outside of the bathtub, my body flattened atop this bench, arms under my shoulders supporting me against the tub rim, and my mother *in* the bathtub holding the extendable showerhead, trying to shampoo and rinse my hair for the first time in weeks. This was a comedy skit that I will cherish forever. It is also possible to enrobe kitchen plastic wrap around your torso and take a speedy shower, use a cape from a hair salon (or cut a hole in a plastic garbage bag) to keep your shoulders and back dry, go outside to the cold garden hose, or leverage a combination of such creative options. Should you be allowed to replace your bandage with a fresh one, be extra sure there is no air, dirt, or water under the bandage. Like I keep saying, you'll figure it all out because you'll have to! Plus, the incentive of feeling like yourself again after a good shower and real shampoo is a hefty one!

A teeny perk to sneak in here for the patient: You will have minions to acquire, cook, and (if you're lucky) serve you food. Don't get too used to it, but relish being served a tray of food on a pillowy throne while you can. You're in no state to cook anyway, between the pain, the drugs, and the lack of appetite. If your minions are not chefs, stock up on pre-made food ahead of time. Maybe your work or school will organize a "meal train" to deliver homemade meals to you for a few days. This will be short-lived, and once you're independently mobile again, you should use these activities to set teeny tiny goals for yourself throughout the day. It's important to push yourself a little bit at a time to keep progressing and strengthening. Just be sure to avoid bending, lifting, and twisting as you heal.

Incentive spirometer

Most people may never need to know what this is, but you may be a lucky one who finds out. Don't worry, it's nothing scary.

After surgery, your back hurts and you're not exactly inclined to cough or take deep breaths. Cue the incentive spirometer. The cutest and simplest device to coax you into taking slow, deep breaths to inflate the lungs and prevent pneumonia. It's essentially a plastic mouthpiece connected by a tube to a chamber with a little ball in it. The goal is to use your breath to float the ball up higher and higher. (There are printed numbers along the side to track progress.) Blowing against some resistance forces you to inflate your lungs.

Do *not* get discouraged if those little numbers seem impossible to hit. You *will* eventually re-expand your lungs to the point where you can take deep, rejuvenating breaths. Like all good things, this will take time and practice, so take it easy on yourself and keep the spirometer on hand throughout the day (even though it is one more annoyance you may not want to tolerate when in pain and on drugs). Your cardiovascular system has been through a lot lately; view this little plastic object as your friend!

The post-op poop

Between the hospital food, volume of medications, inactivity, change in routine, and overall stress on your body and mind, there's plenty to back you up. If your surgery includes some lumbar incision, then don't be surprised if there's also a lack of muscular assistance. (There are muscles in your lower back and surrounding area that contribute to help you poop, which is made very clear when you can't contract any of them.)

It's to be expected. Stock up on laxatives for your recovery phase, and ask your doctor if you should take them in advance of the surgery day too. Your muscles *will* regain strength and everything will go back to normal.

Re-learning basic life tasks

Your post-op world may take some getting used to. This is something I *wish* had been explained to me when I was about to undergo surgery, and I've heard that wish echoed from other warriors. Ahead are some situations compiled from fusioneers, but you are sure to have your own unique experiences and encounter your own puzzles. Just take it easy and know that we *all* go through a similar process. You weren't born knowing how to dress yourself or drive a car; these had to be learned. Now you just need to learn how to adjust these "basic life tasks" to suit your new and improved body, "re-learning" them, in a sense.

Let's begin with getting out of bed in the morning. Never mind hitting the snooze alarm or having to be alert before the sun; getting out of the bed in itself will need some work. Pre-op you may have been able to legitimately bounce out of bed, sitting straight up and swinging your legs over the edge to face the day. Not so anymore, my little post-op acorn. Regardless of your fusion level, a portion of you is now largely immobile and may still be sore. That means that when you go to sit up directly, you are hauling that section of you up without any contributing effort on its part. This is going to put strain on the surrounding areas if you continue your pre-op method without adjusting.

The hospital team will teach you to roll onto one side, scoot to the edge of the bed facing out, and place your upper hand against the mattress to push yourself up slowly into a seated position. From there, just stand up. The same is going to be true for getting horizontal. Sit first, then lay yourself down slowly using your hands as supports. You are bound to find a way of getting out of bed in the morning that works for *you*. After a while, it becomes second nature.

Next up: getting dressed. Once again, this will depend on the fusion location and pain levels of the day. The mobility issue that really took me by surprise, though, was putting on pants. What a simple task to tackle, right? That's what I thought too! I would try every morning, once I was mobile again, to put on pants. Each time resulted in a different experience in frustration. It seemed ridiculous that a simple task I used to do every day of my life was now so complicated. Lift? Bend? One foot? How do I reach my ankle? How can *anybody* wear pants?

Eventually I had to ask for a demo. Lounging around with one of my friends in her room a few months post-op, we were looking at new items in her fashionista closet. She threw on a new pair of jeans and something clicked in my head. "I know this sounds like a ridiculous request," I said, "but I can't remember how to put pants on anymore and keep falling over myself. It's like I can't reach... something? Could you just remind me? Please?" Bless her, she grabbed another pair of pants and put them on, bending forward in an easy arch to step into one leg hole at a time, balancing on the other leg in-between. Remaining arched, she slid them up and, *ta-da*, done! "Ah-ha!" I said in a new moment of clarity. "I no longer have that forward arch-ability and my balance has entirely changed. That explains it!" We laughed about it, and I went home to devise a new method to don pants.

Immediate solution: Place your butt against a wall or chair to take care of the balance issue. No shame in added stability! Bring your knees up to you rather than bending down, and pull the pants up bit by bit instead of hopping into them. Or just wear skirts for a bit.

Now that we are fully clothed, let's address the kindergarten skill of putting on and lacing up your shoes. Cheat with Velcro and slip-on shoes as much as you like, but eventually you will need to address laces once again. We've established that full back bending is no longer a feature offered in this vessel (especially during the first few months post-op when you *must* avoid any bending). From now on, you will be folding at the knees to get to your footwear! This can be a quick low squat to grab your shoes from the floor, or you can store footwear in a higher rack to have them on hand. As for getting them on, one method is to pull your feet up one at a time *to your torso* using your hands (as opposed to bringing your torso *to your feet*) while sitting on a chair or on the ground, or leaning against a wall. Then place the shoe onto the foot and lace it up. Your method of choice will likely depend on the location and type of surgery, but you *will* develop your own style to get it done.

An absolute two-in-one frustration is trying to tie shoes while confined to a seated position in a car, train, plane, or bus. You have nowhere to stretch your leg to bring it *in* to you (instead of going *to* it) or space on either side to swing your fused torso. You are in a mime's invisible box of titanium fusion, where your *only* option for reaching those laces is forward and down. Feeling like a T-Rex with arms way too short to be any good, you bend over the seatbelt at your waist, digging your face into the seat back or dash in front of you. "Ah! Why can't I reach?! So. Close. Please!" Once again, deep breath. Use your hands to bring one foot up to the edge of the seat, where you should be able to prop your heel and get a handle on your laces. At that point, you have also likely entertained all the passengers around you. Get creative if you absolutely have to lace up while seated… otherwise, wait until you get to stand up or move. Remember that shoelaces aren't exactly mission critical as a passenger.

"I see your car shoes and raise you car ski boots." Okay, ante up! Should you happen to be a downhill skier, you know all too well how those plastic foot cages are tough to put on in a spacious ski chalet *without* a fusion. I trust you can imagine how limited your space will become in a car cab *with* a fusion restricting your range of motion, not to mention wrestling those metal clasps shut all the way to the toes. If you have gotten used to quickly putting your ski boots on in the passenger seat of a warm car with the doors closed, know that suiting up in the car with the doors shut is not going to be such an easy time-saver anymore.

You will figure all of this out for yourself. Consider this just a friendly "heads up" that the way things "used" to be done may no longer be available… and that we all adapted quite quickly.

Return-to-school prep

After surgery, after home recovery, school will come back into play. Yet again, it's best to prepare for this chapter *in advance*. Your surgeon will have a rough recovery timeline for you to work with, completely dependent on your situation. It's advisable to notify the school's administration of the surgery date and recovery timeline so you can make a plan together. You will be absent for a few weeks, and teachers will likely be ready to help however they can. But be *honest* with them about your estimated recovery timeline – you won't be ready for homework right away! Some warriors didn't have to submit some assignments or tests. Others got additional tutoring from the teachers to catch up on the course material. In any case, your time recovering in hospital should not be spent thinking about school *at all*, and your return should go fairly smoothly.

You're also not the first student at your school to ever have a surgery, so the staff likely already have some ideas for accommodations. Maybe your first week back can just be half days. If there's an elevator, they can lend you the key so you can avoid stairs and crowds. Ask to leave class a bit earlier to avoid being jostled in hallway crowds. Is there a nurse's office or prayer room of some sort? You can get access to that if you're in pain and just need a break to recharge. Maybe even gain access to ice packs or heating pads – the area around your incision is likely to still feel tingly, numb, and strange.

Carrying heavy backpacks full of books is *out of the question*. (Remember, no bending, lifting, or twisting.) Can they coordinate some book buddies to help you through the hallways if your friends have completely different classes? Maybe a second set of textbooks to leave at home? Bending down or reaching up to high lockers is also not welcome. Is there a better locker or more convenient locker location you could be given? Speaking of uncomfortable things, school chairs are not exactly cushy recliners. Get permission to leave a pillow in each of your classrooms so you don't have to carry one all around with you.

There are tons of potential accommodations and the school *wants* you to succeed. You just have to begin by *asking*! Talk to your surgeon as well – they probably have more ideas to share from all of their other patients over the years!

If you have a favorite sport that you absolutely want to get back into ASAP, be honest with your surgeon about it so they can bake it into your recovery plan. A spinal fusion can accommodate most activities, but you will *not* be rushing back into all sports immediately. Take one day at a time, and share this part of your recovery plan with the school or coaches to clear up any gym class questions.

Some patients only miss a few weeks of school and are back to their regular activities in as little as four months; some take longer. *Every patient experience is different*, but a positive and determined mindset plays a huge role.

No more regular radiation

No more regular radiation doses. No more regular hospital appointments. On to learning how to care for yourself and your new back for the long haul!

P.S. No. Multiple X-rays per year will not radiate you to the point of getting superpowers. Radiation still isn't that good for you, though. Thankfully we live in an exciting time where low-radiation X-ray technologies are being developed.

Ask your doctor if there is such a machine nearby that you could use instead of traditional X-ray machines. It also doesn't hurt to check regularly for signs of thyroid or breast cancer if you are regularly being exposed to radiation.[34]

"Cured"? Okay, back to "normal" now!

Once your surgery is done and healed, the world may expect you to bounce back into "normal" society again. Just like that. After all, you're "cured" now and ready to face the real world!

But wait... you've never been in that world before. You were in a slightly different world filled with appointments, adjustments, plastic shells, and imbalances – and you had no metal in you. It's like scoliosis was a type of crutch you always had (you were leaning a bit to one side, after all) and that crutch has all of a sudden been kicked out from under you. It can feel like you barely had the time to relearn how to walk before it's time to fly! Not to mention a spinal fusion is not a "cure."

You're not alone. We all want to slowly ease back into life and get our bearings before jumping back into the "real" world once again. And so we should.

Know that that kind of readjustment does *not* happen overnight, even though people may expect it to. You may be extra surprised to get that kind of push from your parents of all people! But when you think about their point of view, it kind of makes sense. They've spent years watching you grow in pain, maybe dealing with braces and undergoing invasive surgery. They're ready for that chapter to end and for your "real" life to begin! Trying to push you forward into this new world is a natural way for them to try and leave the *ow* behind (for you and for them).

So how can we, as scolis, handle this? Well, let me say this: If bracing or waiting for surgery was ever an excuse to limit your activities, that excuse is gone now. Your time in the brace is over; your surgery is complete. Now you move on with your life mindfully aware that, although people may seem to push you, *you need not rush*. Step into your future at *your* pace. Be slower with yourself, take rests (especially fresh after surgery), but push yourself a bit more each day. It's way easier if you motivate yourself, rather than somebody else telling you what to do. Let's also remind ourselves that scoliosis cannot be "cured"; it is only "managed"... it is still very much with you.

Your post-op experience may seem to drop you on your own into this "new" world without ongoing care from your past medical team. You may even feel somewhat abandoned. But it's time to move on and create your *new* medical support system around you, moving onto *your* new normal.

The Scoliosis Journey with a Fusion

Many, many, many questions arise about spinal fusion and life with rods. While we will not go into details about different back operations, methods, scientific statistics, and all of that nitty gritty stuff, we *will* take a look at "real people" experiences and perspectives. Most come with tips that can make fused restrictions so much easier. Not to mention the hilarity that can ensue from being fused.

Here is what real life with spinal fusion surgery can look and feel like.

AROUND THE HOUSE

Toilet paper dispenser location

Who the heck actually wants their toilet paper roll mounted to the wall *behind* the toilet? Who? Certainly there is only a minimal subset of the population who can actually reach it without insult or injury. Our own little group, for example, has limited ability to twist and turn, especially from a seated position.

Some bathrooms may only have space available behind the can to install the TP dispenser. Okay, fair, it's necessary, we get it. But what about the designs where there is plenty of wall space *around* the throne and yet the designer made a *conscious decision* to put the dispenser around back. Absolutely zero user experience consideration given there.

I suspect this is "one of those things" you don't think about until it happens to you. You locate it once you're ready to make use of the paper supply, go to reach for it, only to realize that your spine doesn't twist that way and your shoulder muscles are not willing to cooperate. Well, sh!t.

This nuisance was made starkly evident to me in my own apartment, which had such a foolish setup. The loo had a very nice wall on one side that was begging for a TP dispenser, but instead it was installed on the back wall almost touching the reservoir. Now *that* is too far back. After the first few attempts of feeling like an invalid, unable to reach the darn thing, I began simply leaving the TP rolls on top of the counter within reach.

Now hear this, interior designers and builders, put yourselves in our shoes and pop yourself onto the throne. Where are you able to reach with little to no torso movement? Good. Now install the dispenser there and stop making us squirm.

Bathtubs

I took a journey to an empty standard-issue bathtub with my laptop for you all, dear readers. Here I sit, fully clothed, computer perched on my knees, increasingly uncomfortable by the millisecond. I'll write this quickly so that we can all get out of here.

What most folks consider a leisurely activity, the bubble bath is no true friend to this lumbar fusioneer. First of all, a basic bathtub is hard and rectangular. There's a cavernous space between my straight fused back and the straight hard back of the tub, each sitting at very different slopes, neither about to curve or concede. This fused spine will not smoothly conform to the shape of the bathtub, leaving all connections between the body and bath up to the tip and tail. It certainly doesn't help that hard tubs have no mushy parts for comfort against the tailbone, prominences, or shoulder wing. (Note that a synonym for "hard" happens to be "backbreaking.") That's not usually an issue for dry seating options – we can always readjust, comfortably using supports and fluffy pillows. But we're not about to make the bathtub cushiony and supportive since adding couch cushions to a tub full of water is not exactly going to go well.

If you sit upright, your lower half is warmly immersed in soapy water but your torso is above the water line and growing colder by the second. Time to dunk your entire body underwater to capture that supposedly relaxing feeling!

You *slide* yourself down by bending the knees, the back of your neck coming to rest against the top edge, feeling the bubbles tickle your chin. *Ooh*, this could totally be relaxing! Lavender candle and some music on, let's just soak it all in and add some Epsom salts.

Tailbone grinding against the bottom. *Ow*. Readjust. Shoulder blades crunching against the back ridge. *Ow*. Readjust. Back of the neck and head do not like the hard rim of the tub; that's going to bruise. Let's try lying on one side instead. *Ow*. Readjust. Hip bone having a fight with the ceramic. *Ow*. Readjust. Let's sit up and give our edges a break... and now we're cold again.

Rigid + rigid does not always play well together. So, what can we do? Well, instead of renovating an entire room to fit an entirely new bathtub that has slopes, seats, or curves that your back *may* rest more comfortably against, let's go for the quick wins! Bathtub pillows can be purchased that can take some of the direct impact off of the neck, head, and tailbone. Some dry out better than others, so read the reviews. You can spend less time in the bath, limiting the amount of times you have to readjust and reimmerse yourself. If your goal in a tub is simply to be surrounded by heat for a while, hot tubs are a great option since the bathers are immersed much deeper to keep warm! While certainly not for washing, they create far less pressure on the tip and tail since there are *real* seats molded into them.

It is now time to get out of this bath. To get the full experience, I did not use any towels or pillows to cushion my angles while sitting here writing in a dry tub. Tortured artist, indeed. *Ow*.

Making beds

The laundry, the folding, the unfolding, the reaching, the bending, the fusion, the tucking, the smoothing... lots goes into making a bed! Notice how the above equation includes "the fusion"? Making a bed is still very much a part of the household duties list, and a fusion does not prevent it. It can just make it look a little different.

Imagine taping a long ruler down your back, and then going to make the bed. Here's hoping you have a single bed! There may be some steep bending at the waist to smooth out the center of the bed sheet in lieu of curving forward. You may not be able to side-bend into a tricky corner where the fitted sheet needs help, requiring instead that you crawl *onto* the bed to tackle that section.

You may have to get into a deep squat to lift that mattress edge so as to avoid lifting it with a flattened back and straining. (Lifting the edges of king-size mattresses has hurt me when I wasn't being careful.)

There's no rush here, so watch your core and support yourself on your arms if needed as you cross this chore off the list. Making beds is not a competition, but if it were, you could win just on the creativity points alone.

Gardening

Bending down low to toil in the soil for hours on end? *Ow*. If you must, set small goals and time limits with breaks to stand and stretch.

Wanting to stretch between your vertebrae

Oh, how I long for that feeling. But there will never again be any stretching movement between those fused vertebrae… at times frustratingly so.

Hot rod fevers

You know how your muscles and bones ache when you have the flu? Hopefully you rarely get illnesses that are accompanied by a fever, but should you catch some such germ it *might* feel like a fever around your hardware. A fever within a fever.

Squirm as you may, just like the rest of the flu there's no escaping it. This may also be the only time that you ever *feel* your rods (or think you do). It may feel like the rods are heating up, but nothing of the sort is going to happen – *you* are just heating up because of a fever. Endure it, let the illness run its course, and wait it out – that's the only combination cure here. Flu medicine can dull the senses a bit, which any non-fusion person would take anyway. This too shall pass. Sleep it off and drink plenty of fluids.

By the way, you can play this to your advantage. Now that you know what that feeling is and what it means, you'll recognize it as an early warning sign that you have some virus. Brace for impact and go buy flu meds.

Note: Some fusioneers say they can feel the cold in their hardware when they go outside on very frosty days.

OUT AND ABOUT

Shoulder checking in cars

Take note: Spinal fusion affects your ability to twist (not just bend). Many of us are surprised by the extent of this, especially when we go to drive a car – and *especially* if we need to learn to drive after the fusion.

My driving instructor was a sweet older man who had seen just about everything in that job. Apparently, he had never seen a fusioneer try to shoulder check for the first time, though. About six months post-op, I tried my best – which was apparently torquing my *entire* body from head to pelvis, taking the steering wheel with me – to look behind me before changing lanes. That's a heck of a big shoulder check! A true teacher, he took his time to help me simply cast a glance over my shoulder.

Take it easy going back to driving after surgery. Take the time to get used to your body's new range of motion in an empty parking lot first.

Small cars = small door frames

Should you be an unfused tall person, you're already used to bumping your head on doors frames, car visors, and low light fixtures. How about after you've had a spinal fusion and your ability to curve down to duck is restricted? *Ow*.

About a year after recovery, I went shopping for a new car. Just something simple to zip around town that wasn't outrageously priced. The salesman said, "That's not a problem. I have a used compact car that just came in with low mileage and a low price tag." Excellent! It looked good from the outside, so I went on to try the seats. Well, well, well... bit of a problem here! I could *not* get into the driver's seat. The door frame was too small! I kept trying and trying, but I just kept bonking my head on the upper rim. I had to get out, hinge at the hips to fold my torso forward, and dive head-first into the car to clear the door frame. Once inside it was mockingly comfortable with lots of legroom. "Okay," I remember thinking to myself, "pretty decent once inside, and I figured out how to get *in* so I could live with this. Now let's try out the back seats for my passengers."

Just when we thought the show was over, I implemented my new forward-bend attack to get into the *back* seat. Equally comfy back there, this was looking like an acceptable car! My search may be over, and so quickly! Now it was time to get out of the car and give it a more thorough once-over. I mentally psyched myself up: "Get out of the car." *Bonk.* "Okay, get out of the car." *Bonk.* "Come on, woman, just bend down and clear the door frame here." *Bonk.* "Stop hitting your head!" The salesman didn't know *what* was going on. "Okay, one more try." *Bonk.* "Arghhh!" I was stuck in the backseat of that tiny car and could not get out. I was still fairly fresh to my new permanently poised position, and my movement education was still underway.

Think it's just me? Think again. When I ask fusioneers about "weird" things that happen to them due to their fusions, I mention small car doors as an example. Their face always goes from ponderous to instant recognition. "*Ohhh* yeah! Hah! That *always* happens to me still." Years post-op, it is still all too easy to forget to roll your neck sideways before getting into and out of cars. *Thwack.* There she goes again. Don't even get me started on coaxing a fusion into the back seat of a two-door car.

Learn to move slowly when getting in and out of cars to save your noggin from hitting the frame. Sometimes you'll need to lean forward to *dive* into a car, and other times you may need to lean *way* back and limbo out of the seat (which I eventually figured out to escape the backseat of that car I did *not* end up buying). This is entirely self-paced learning. Nobody else is in your body or knows how you're feeling, so it's up to you. Deep breath, take it slow... you got this.

A side note: Some people who do not know you are fused – or worse, clueless people who know you are fused but are unthinking clods – may laugh at you when you hit your head on the door frame. They don't consider your world when you encounter "simple" obstacles from their world. I have personally heard "Ha-ha, dummy, just bend to avoid the door frame!" Well, I *can't!* Own it, ignore it, or work on avoiding frames more... Your call about how to address it. Just know that you're not alone, and it hurts way more than it is funny.

Vehicle seating

If you don't find car seats comfortable, you're not the only one. What were the car manufacturers thinking when they designed these new and improved "safer seats" in vehicles? The lower back and shoulder/neck pain they cause can feel like you're being pushed and pulled in every wrong direction. When you add in the angle of the steering wheel or the pedals locking your legs into one formation, it's anything *but* a comfy cruise.

"These new seat designs and head-rest angles provide better impact in the event of an accident! They're the latest technology! See how well my non-fused body fits in this seat and where the impact will go should I hit something?" Sorry, car salesman, you are not selling me on this at *all*. Watch *me* sit in this seat: My fused back is unsupported by the backrest and my neck is forced sharply downwards by the headrest. Where is that ever-so-important lumbar support, at a minimum? I have no flexibility to melt into this seat design. My pre-formed body is clashing with it in the most unnatural shape possible. Don't have a sales pitch for that, now do ya?

Let's acknowledge that not every consumer good is made to suit everybody. Thankfully in recent years, the headrest tilt has been lessened noticeably from the initial over-aggressive design. Maybe they're working their way up to making headrests and seat shapes personally adjustable too! (Wishful thinking.)

We do have to hand it to the car designers who introduced heated seats as a common feature. Turning that bad boy on high can warm up the lumbar nicely while in motion! A little soothing treat for the lower back. Now can they build that in for the neck and shoulders too?

The world may not be designed with us in mind, but that just means we need to come up with our own designs and share our best practices. What can we do when car seats reduce us to tears? Place a small pillow between your back and the backrest to instantly lessen those strains. It's just as easy to ball up a coat or scarf to serve as temporary support (same for airplanes and trains). After all, you need to be safe when operating a vehicle, and being distracted by teeth-grinding discomfort is not a great idea.

If you also can't twist in the front seat to quickly grab something out of the back seat, well... get out of the car to go get it. We have yet to find a scoli life hack for that!

Hardware science

You are not a lightning rod. In the full-disclosure spirit of this book, I did not think about this until my first outing in a thunderstorm post-surgery. If you weren't scared of lightning storms before, you don't need to be now.

While we're talking about metallic properties, you will not be able to stick fridge magnets to your back. (Yes, I tried this post-op.) Additionally, your rods will not set off the metal detectors at airports, buildings, or events. I have never been pulled aside by airport security because of them.

Spooky "new" pains

Once in a while, some new spot of pain may present itself around your fused back. Depending on the way your brain handles pain, you may pay it little to no mind or you may perk up at its appearance. You may freeze on the spot to do a quick self-scan by touch, searching for anything numb, sharp, out of the ordinary... Okay, now slowly try to move... analyzing... stand up straight... feel for any heat... nothing terrible? Oh, it's fine? Okay, cool, great. Off we go with the rest of our day!

Experiencing different kinds of pain is almost a game. Like a roulette wheel where slivers of the wheel get replaced periodically to keep it entertaining. Some muscular discomfort, some structural clicks, a deep ache, a sudden sharp pain, muscle knots in a smattering of locations, tension you just need to walk off, or a pain that calls for lying horizontal... such variety! And they can happen at any time when sitting too long, raising your arms too high, misstepping, lifting something heavy, breathing...

The post-op recovery phase of muscles and nerves settling down is particularly fascinating. Many of us have weird tingles, twitches, and pains around our backs during the first year or so after surgery. One fusioneer temporarily experienced a *very* sensitive spot on her lower back that got in the way of sitting down or lying against it. Another fusioneer experienced a bruised feeling under a portion of her ribcage. Other warriors have reported pains in their neck and shoulders that required heat sessions or massage guns every evening. Perhaps the wildest feeling is when a numb post-op back is itchy... your brain knows you're scratching that spot, but the spot doesn't know it, so the ghost itch persists.

All of these new "surprise" sensations in our backs can feel spooky and mysterious. Sometimes our brains like to run worst-case scenarios that some structural damage has happened, distracting us with thoughts of "*Ow*! Oh my heavens, what could this possibly be? Did some of my hardware break?!" Many fusioneers seem to react similarly to new pains: Scan to make sure nothing is broken and do some kind of physical therapy with hot/cold home treatment. (It does happen that rods break or screws come loose, so be sure to speak up if you feel something very wrong. Apparently the sound of a rod breaking is *quite* loud.)

Posture

Unfused warriors often get comments about their "off-center" balance or "poor posture," when in reality, they *are* standing up tall and poised in their scoli form. When a fusion comes into play, there is yet another impact on posture.

Being fused from the center of my back almost to my tailbone, I am ramrod straight. (I guess pun intended.) I just can't help it. Whether I am sitting, standing, or heaven help me lying on the ground while out camping, I am one shape in my center.

So many people tell me they wish they had my good posture. Even though mine is metallically enhanced and full of imbalances, they don't know that. On more than one occasion, strangers have approached me asking if I were a ballerina, especially if my hair was up in a topknot. Should it happen to you as well, thank them kindly and enjoy that compliment buzz for the rest of the week.

If they don't go all the way to "ballerina," they may notice you anyway and use that to train their children. I was once sitting outside on a curb, waiting for a friend, when a lady walked by me with five children in tow. She looked exhausted (completely understandable) and clearly thought I wouldn't hear her when she said to the kids, "See! Look at how good her posture is! You guys should sit like that more often. It's good for you and look how nice she looks. Oh, she heard me! I'm sorry, miss. Ignore me!" That single-sided interaction made me smile then and still does now as I write about it.

Having "perfect posture" all of the time is hard work, though. Bodies want to hang out in their most-energy-efficient configuration possible. With scoliosis, that means relaxing into the pattern the curves have provided *around* the fusion, which does nothing to actively counter the scoli effects. While you can force yourself to hold a posture for a while, eventually your body is going to get tired. Many of us have found PSSE helpful as the course focuses on how to strengthen your own body into a more stable state – not always something that comes easily without a professional guide, since scoli can play tricks on your mind (pre-op and post-op). Time to learn and improve!

As an added bonus in the scoli gift basket you never ordered, we always look like we're paying attention (good for school and work). It also adds a touch of class to a society that is now seeing more and more people slouched over in front of computers and phones. (You should still be aware of "tech neck" from straining forward during too much screen time.) People may not want all of what you have, but there are some perks. Use it to your advantage and build on that poise.

Classes at the gym

Ha! I laugh at you, trainer. There will be no perfect "cat" or "cow" in my cat-cow pose. It ain't happening post-surgery, fused from thoracic to lumbar. Nor will "slowly rolling up one vertebra at a time" from a folded position look all that graceful. It's going to be a slow roll for about three seconds, and then a slow pendulum swing upwards to standing. Sorry (not sorry).

Oftentimes during floor exercises you'll hear the trainer say, "Make sure your back stays flat on the mat! I don't want any arches or holes under your back!" Your PSSE therapist can guide you on how to best support your back during floor exercises, teaching you adjustments you can bring with you to these gym classes.

Lying on your back can cause it to feel quite twisted and angular. And fighting the floor for comfort can get frustrating. If pointy or rotated body parts are rebelling against the hard floor and causing discomfort, support them with padding. I don't always have special pads with me, but I keep a sweater or pair of socks within arm's reach at the gym. Tuck that little bundle of cloth between your body and the mat to get proper support and cushiness. Build in your own comfort!

Eating messy food at a low table

This is a valid nuisance for an adult with a great fusion, let me tell you. You just go ahead and try to pick up a forkful of peas from your plate with a ruler taped to your back. A balancing act is soon to follow as you try your darnedest to retain every roly-poly pea on that fork as it wobbles toward your mouth. That's right, it's all up to the fork, because your *torso* is not going to curve forward to get closer to the table to minimize the disaster scene of your escaped peas falling all over the place!

All those folks with forward-bending spines have the option of leaning in low and gobbling up their wild rice near their plate with no casualties. But not you! Those people simply don't know this is a real, volatile problem for you, so you are left looking like a toddler in need of a bib and a high chair. Additionally, lifting up a fully loaded plate to your mouth with one hand while holding your fork in the other is a balancing act that rarely works out. (Or even worse, a bowl of soup.)

The faster you can move it into your mouth in one swift *swoop*, the less chance that tasty morsel will fall off your spoon/fork/burrito. Alternatively, scoot your chair back as far as you need to lever your face closer to the food zone. This one can easily be filed under "Things Non-Fused People Would Never Consider."

Creating stories

When I was in my early twenties, out with some gal pals late one night, a boy struck up a conversation with me while we were in line for 2:00 a.m. sandwiches. This guy was cute, seemed normal, and even politely held the restaurant doors open for us. He was quite a bit shorter than my six-foot tower, which contributed to his being more eye-level with my back than my face. My evening outfit included a top that exposed my lower back featuring my slim pink scar. This boy turned out to be way less cute when he randomly pointed at my scar and loudly said with a shocked expression, "*Woahhh*, what's that? What happened to your back?"

I could have melted on the spot. I was so horrified that (a) it was apparently *that* noticeable, (b) I was reminded of that medical saga during a night of fun, and (c) if he reacted like that out loud, that must be how other people react internally when they spot it.

Right?

Wrong.

When those thoughts finished passing through my head for about three seconds, I whipped around and said, "Surf trick gone wrong." Now, I'll give the benefit of the doubt that he couldn't have known it would upset me quite that much. But the reality is that an unfortunate number of people have poor manners and everyone handles trauma differently... and those two methods don't mix too well. Basic manners aside, nobody knows what others have gone through and – this is key – not everybody thinks before they speak.

Right from the start, I set limits about how much of my medical history I would share with strangers and used comedy whenever possible. Saying "I had surgery for scoliosis" often warranted more explanation and discussion since so many people didn't know anything about it... or did not actually care to know. While that education is certainly important to spread, sometimes I just don't have the time or energy for it – and sometimes it's 2:00 a.m. and not the right location for an education session. Strangers don't need to be fully aware of what you went through, and you don't need to get into the weeds about it all of the time – unless you *want* to. Your business is your own.

If you're not quite comfortable talking about it yet, that's okay! It took me quite a while to gain that confidence. I sometimes took liberties with more "fun" stories to feed nosy inquirers when they pried. I liked "shark attack" or "wrestled a crocodile" for a succinct response. What's truly important is your self-acceptance and open dialogue with your friends and family – never close yourself off entirely.

The Scoliosis Journey Through Life

Braced, pre-op, post-op, no-op… whether or not you had a brace or surgery, the fact remains that you have (or your loved one has) scoliosis. It goes without saying that scoliosis can be a real pain in the… back. There are bends and curves within that are skewing all kinds of alignments. They can be managed with proper care, support, education, and medication.

Ahead is a compilation of daily activities, emotions, challenges, and personal experiences associated with scoliosis. While you will have your own approaches to some things, you may find new tips, tricks, or perspectives to consider – many of us would have wanted to know all this ahead of time to skip through the frustration of our own solution-seeking. We learn a lot through the experience of scoliosis – maybe more than you've realized – including the importance of taking care of both our mental and physical health.

Each person is completely unique and not everything will apply to you… but you're likely to find something that will make you say, "I thought that was just *me*!" It's uplifting to discover that you're not the only one experiencing something scoli-related that no non-scoli could understand.

Here is what real life with idiopathic scoliosis, with or without surgery, can look and feel like.

OW! WHAT A PAIN IN THE BACK

Pain changes

While many scolis claim to have no pain from scoliosis, others have numerous discomforts courtesy of scoliosis. Many fusioneers have told me that pain is the main reason they chose to have surgery.

For those of us dealing with scoli pain, we know that pain is fluid. It doesn't stay the same every single minute of every single day. Pain keeps you on your toes. It comes, goes, and changes in intensity depending on where pressure is being applied, what activities you did or didn't do, how tired you are, and which stressors are at play.[35] What to do about this pain? Will it go away on its own? Does it just need a nudge? How about some rest? Meds? Are there some brain-calming techniques to learn and apply? But no matter what... pain does exist.

Pain can also be temporary. You learn over time how to best care for your body to give it the exercise, rest, treatment, medication, or meditation time it needs. There are physical and emotional tools out there that have helped many a pain endurer – it might take a bit of searching and faith, and it may not be easy, but it's possible to alleviate many pains.

There is a psychological side to pain: the relationship the person has with the pain. Everything going on within us is so connected and integrated, we don't quite know where the mind ends and the inflammatory agents and cortisone begin. It's important for a psychologist to be there *when* a person has pain.

If you're having a bad day, take stock of your accumulated tips and tricks in your scoli toolkit. You either *know* what you need right now or can *learn* about what else is out there.

Pain is subjective

Where does it hurt? Everywhere. How much does it hurt? A lot. What kind of pain is it? I don't know... the bad kind.

Pain is completely subjective and even your own "pain scale" calibration can change daily. Your pain tolerance and numerous environmental factors will affect how you feel, making it hard to compare apples to apples. Maybe today you woke up feeling like yellow apples. Tomorrow you will feel like furious red apples, and your assessment will be through that lens.

Nobody else is in your shoes, which makes it tough to explain your pain to the professionals to the point they fully, truly, completely understand. Doctors may ask you to keep a medical journal of what activities you do daily and what level of pain you experience. They are sincere in their efforts and really want to help through this data. But even the best judge of your body, *you*, may find it hard to track pain against any specific, static metric.

Be as honest as you can with your doctor and caregivers, even if your view changes daily. Do your part to keep everybody on the same page with a log of your scoliosis "events" and feelings. Your scoli journal doesn't have to be full paragraphs – just a little something that you can use as a point of reference. Get creative with your descriptions if a "1 to 10" scale isn't working for you. Use images or colors to describe how it feels. Here's one from mine: "I can't sit anymore today. My whole lower back feels like a brick on fire and I can't escape it. The muscles are so hard on one side that I look like half a body builder." Taking this seriously and being honest will help ease the worries of your family, your doctors, and yourself.

Apples and appointments aside, it's a good idea to keep some kind of journal for your *own* information. I took some sporadic notes here and there over the years and genuinely wish I had done it more consistently. Looking back, there were many "back incidents" I wouldn't mind reading about for an indication of what I did to help get through them and how I felt at the time. It's all too easy to forget a bad event in your life, move on, and then feel lost when it happens again.

If you already have your own "pain scale" and/or medical journal on the go, way to go!

Sitting for a long time

Some scolis love to walk for a long time and can't stand sitting. Others love to sit and can't stand long walks.

Sitting is my number-one nemesis… the reason I think all-inclusive resorts or cottage weekends with friends where "we'll just sit around and do nothing, it'll be great!" will actually be terrible. The reason I am always walking around the block, making my neighbors suspect I'm casing the joint. The reason I can walk 20 minutes to a grocery store and then back again without thinking it's foolish. The reason I don't want to watch two-hour-plus movies without an intermission. The reason board game nights don't float my boat. The reason I'm sometimes late to a dinner because I walked there, much to some friend's ridicule and lack of understanding. The reason I dream about sitting and doing nothing for once without paying for it for the next two days.

"Sitting can't hurt a back if it's not moving or straining, right?" Not quite. Sitting allows your body to naturally sink into the shape it wants... which is not always what's best. Casually relaxing into your curves is not doing anything to actively counter them.[36] It also turns out that the discs in your spine take on more load while you're sitting than standing.[37]

Extensive sitting and giving in to your curves may be something you don't realize is happening until you're *too* aware of it. Let's burst those doors wide open here. Think about all the casual reasons you sit throughout a normal day: studying, using public transportation, driving, watching TV, playing video games, eating, reading, socializing. And what about the sitting where you have no say in the duration or type of seating? Planes, trains, waiting rooms, lectures, work offices, conferences, hair salon chairs, nail salon chairs, veterinary offices, sports venues... lots of sitting opportunities! Oh, those are all great fun.

Life as a human requires sitting, and on occasion for long periods of time. Be mindful of your posture and curves – you'll be doing yourself a favor! If you're not sure how to adjust properly *for your spine*, contact a PSSE therapist. Invest in a zero gravity chair for your outdoor lounging time to recline in comfort with a book in the sun. Get supports like armrests and pillows for your office chair. Bring a little lumbar pillow to your hair stylist appointment.

Taking breaks from sitting is wonderfully helpful in alleviating pains and pressures. But what if you don't *want* to take a break? What if you are super in the zone in whatever you are working on? What if you are about to have a breakthrough in your studies? Or maybe you have a tough client meeting and are just about to get them on your side?

Your best-laid plans don't always work out. Yet again, it comes down to a choice you have to make for yourself given the circumstances: "time" versus "situation" versus "pain." Are there consequences to powering through? Are there consequences to stepping away for a moment? It's entirely your call.

Maybe this will cheer you up if you're in pain: taking a few minutes every half hour will make you more productive since you won't be distracted by pain.[38]

Turns out the *ow* doesn't need to get in the way of your productivity, after all! Not only is it good to get the blood flowing, but your eyes will love you if you've been sitting in front of a screen. Your whole body will appreciate a little break.

Standing for a long time

"Sitting for a long time hurts? Okay, well then just stand for a long time instead!"

Unfortunately, scoli life is not quite that simple. It has multidimensional complexities and the sitting/standing equation is no exception. Whether sitting or standing, being in the same position for too long loads weight on the same parts of the spine.[39] It's hard to say if sitting or standing hurts more, as a general rule…

I am bent left and right, rotated front and back, and my sagittal plane is not ideal. This can add up to feeling like a lost little sailboat, leaning my mast in any direction to find pain-free balance, still getting battered by the pain waves as other muscles try to compensate and catch up. Everything gets tired, justifiably so.

I feel immensely better when moving, like on long walks. Prolonged stop-and-go standing, such as browsing stores or museums, was always my undoing. My sailboat kept adjusting and readjusting, weighing anchor only to drop it again, pain permeating deep into my muscles. As yet another joke foisted upon me by the universe, my parents consist of a fashionista and a history buff. Can you see the irony here? The preferred family activities growing up were shopping and going to museums. Since I was constantly ready to go home, it appeared that I had no interest in these events. What we had not yet identified back then was that my dislike of these activities was not so much the content but, rather, the physical discomfort within. Nothing was being visibly *done* to me, but the invisible imbalances deep down were protesting *vehemently*.

Lots of bodies like taking breaks from standing, and ours are no exception. Until we teach those sailboats more stability, here are some warriors' top tips for "too much standing":

- Not only bored people at museums need to "take a load off" and sit once in a while. Look out for empty security guard seats or wide-rimmed plant pots that you can rest your gravity-ridden body on.

- Art galleries and clothing stores often have little couches tucked away in corners. These hidden gems are plentiful once you start looking for them.
- Use footrests or curbs to change up which muscles are activated via your legs.
- Time your arrival at concerts and shows so you won't have to stand around waiting for a long time.
- Pack painkillers just in case the situation becomes too tough to manage.
- If you are truly out of options, endure as best you can, knowing full well you're not breaking any vital structures within. (Don't let your spirit break either.)

You can still handle standing, but learning your comfort limits and taking breaks to make it more pleasant can help. Knowledge is power and, at the end of the day, it's up to *you* to educate yourself on your own body. Talk with specialists to align, balance, and stabilize your sailboat.

Horizontal for a long time

As much as getting a break from the compression of sitting by moving around is very good and necessary, we can't be in motion 24/7... that's simply not possible! Getting horizontal for just a bit and pausing the downward pressure of gravity on our vertebrae is *also* a good thing.

Lying down on your bed at the end of the day, letting your body stretch in each direction, taking a deep breath or two... feeling those little stretches, hearing those little *pops*. All kinds of mini muscles letting go of the day's efforts. It's a unique kind of bliss. You may even luck out and get a good *crack* deep within your back when you're not expecting it. (I used to love these pre-fusion.)

Resting is not "doing nothing." It is doing something: resting!

Just make sure it's not for hours on end – we don't want to have to undo the undo!

If there's "too much" horizontal time, you won't necessarily feel you've done anything "wrong" until you get up. Then the realization that you surpassed your acceptable amount of horizontal time and were immobile for too long crashes over you. You should have known better. (Hello, guilt.) You were lying *in* your curve pattern and now one of your hips is less than an inch away from the bottom of that rib cage.

But wait, how do you know how long "too long" is? Alas, there is no chart available to find your allotted horizontal couch time for your height, weight, and curves. The trick here is to find that fine balance between movement and rest. Exercise is still important for your overall health – don't be a couch potato. At the same time, allow yourself time to relax. Your back should realistically not prevent you from doing what you want to do, but *all in moderation*.

Lie down on the couch, but be aware of your concavities. Watch some TV without being in a seated or standing position. Then change it up!

Long days without stretching

School and employment provide amazing opportunities to learn, earn, socialize, and sometimes even travel! But why oh why is casual stretching still not accepted? Why must schools and employment restrict our freedom of movement, prohibiting us from stretching whenever we want? I'm sure the short answer is "it's not proper." We certainly can't have a solo scoli-yoga session in a lecture hall or office full of cubicles.

Sitting in a lecture hall or conference room, you may swear time slows down when you hurt. Dismissal time never seems to arrive. You just want to leave your restrictive seat and go home to your living room floor for a big ol' stretch! Recall that human spines get loaded more from long periods of sitting than standing.[40] Look at any other animal around you. Your cat/dog/rabbit stretches throughout the day to limber up and counter the constant pressure of gravity. Even birds fluff out their wings and have a li'l stretch. We should too! Alas, such are the facts of life. No serious studying was ever accomplished while stretching on exercise balls during study hall hours. No big business deals were ever signed with the main party away from the conference room doing Pilates. Long days are bound to happen.

How to get around this? There are ways...

Grab some stretch time in between meetings! Take the pre-scheduled breaks during conferences to walk around the hallways or outdoors. Even simpler, use those breaks to go to the washroom and grab a great big arms-in-the-air stretch in the stall (hoping nobody else is in there to see arms coming up over or under the stall, suggesting you're apparently doing something weird on the can). Take the wheelchair stall if you have to – more space for hip rotations! People might give you the dirty eye for taking the wheelchair stall when you clearly don't have a wheelchair, but they're likely also the ones who would look at you sideways if you had a great big stretch in front of the sinks. Park your judgment, folks. People were made to *move*!

Maybe you don't have any space or breaks in your busy day. Let's simplify this once more: Stand up during meetings. Scope out the room and seating layout quickly (in advance, if possible) and pick a chair that has space around it for standing. Make sure your spot is not at the front of a presentation room, where standing would distract everybody and draw attention. Aim for the back center chair; it's no distraction to others and provides the option to stand behind the chair, should the need present itself.

Not at work yet? Don't worry, school is actually easier for this. Even though you aren't exactly allowed to get up and move in the middle of a high school class to un-kink your back, you *can* start with a visit to the administration office or guidance counselor. They can work with you to provide support and ways to refocus on your studies instead of on your pain. In college/university, there is usually an entire department that helps accommodate all types of limitations and disabilities. On both fronts, the school administrators *want* you to succeed and have years of experience helping with all kinds of medical situations. You're not the first, and you won't be the last.

Schools can also provide exam support. Some have separate rooms booked for students who need some kind of accommodation, allowing a lumbar pillow or granting extra time for standing/walking breaks within the room. Makes sense, doesn't it? You need time to move, and however many minutes you need to use in "moving time" is added on to the standard exam time as "lost time." Fair is still fair! Given that exams can be three to four hours long, this is a scoli lifesaver. It also avoids the ginormous gymnasium room exam sessions, where a big stretch or walk could certainly cause a flurry of cheating claims. Look into it and use what's available!

Stepping into a surprise dip in the ground

What a beautiful day to be out for a walk outside, cruising down the sidewalk, enjoying the fresh air, till *BOOM* pothole. *Ow. Owwwww.*

Looking up at the pretty blue sky for a minute while walking can be a mistake when one of your feet plods right into a dip in the ground quite unexpectedly. Thank goodness your ankle doesn't sprain, but it certainly goes down that extra inch or so without your brain knowing in advance. Your knee, hip, lower back, and shoulder all suddenly dip down that extra inch along with it! In a mere millisecond, you sent an impact down one side of your body while your other side tries to catch up. You scan, scan, scan. Ankle doesn't hurt, the hip is upset but it'll calm itself down quickly, back is completely intact but a little shook up, your fusion is angry but it'll get over it. Okay, I think we're good to go. Let's continue this walk and watch where we step from now on!

Surprise impact shocks that reverberate from your foot to your shoulder through your back are *not* listed under the definition of "a pleasant stroll outside."

The weird noises and cracks

Click, thunk, pop, grrrind, kaklunk. Choose your instrument for the scoliorchestra! A hip rotation here for a bass drum, a mini backbend there for a tom or two, a shoulder roll for a snare drum. Maybe you also have a cowbell in your mix. I don't know. Just pray there are no cymbals… those would likely be "bad news" noises.

Most people are used to cracking their knuckles or neck for some instant release. I even have a friend who cracks her nose daily; otherwise, she says it "feels wrong." It's totally "normal" to do this, even though it might gross some people out.

However, there have been *very* mixed reactions to the scoliorchestra. Parents can be mystified, saddened, and concerned by the noises deep within. There are the friends who think it's super cool and always want a hug to see if they can feel what's moving in the back and shoulders. They are mystified by the rarity and mystery!

Then there are the people who *loathe* it. They reveal themselves quickly when you inadvertently crack some tension out of your hips, back, or shoulders while seated next to them. They visibly startle and ask, "What was that? It sounded *deep*!" their eyes wide with concern and revulsion. Yes, that was the orchestra. No, nothing's broken. Don't worry about it.

We could definitely do without these portable scoliorchestras, but *every* body makes noise.

Feeling ancient

Ever feel like you're 90 years old when you're only 20? It may have you considering investing in a walker today that will last you the rest of your life.

Some websites claim most cases of AIS are pain-free, but for those of us who are in pain, we sure know how to "do it up right." When the super painful days pop up, they make you question life in a way that people without chronic pain could never imagine. Your past can pop up: "How did I get here? Has it hurt this bad before?" The possibilities of your future can come soaring in: "If I hurt this much now, what kind of pain will I be in when I'm 90? What will wheelchairs look like in the future?" Most importantly, your present may demand, "What can I do about this today?"

While mobility aids can certainly come in handy, let's not get carried away here... it's all too easy to continue on that choo-choo train of planning for the unknown. You can get derailed if you go too far.

Some days trying to move your body may seem like trying to convince a sack of cement mix to move, except the bag has hardened... and it's cemented to the ground... with a cinder block on top of it. Maybe you slept weird. Maybe you lifted something too heavy. Maybe you sat for too long with your legs crossed... or anything equally random. Or maybe you didn't do anything odd at all and your misalignments simply decided, "That's enough. Let's go on strike. Fire up all pain signals!"

I've had to take sick leave from work for such flare-ups. Initially I tried pushing myself to go to work, thinking that being somewhere busy with lots of distractions would distract me from the pain. Instead, I just squirmed in office chairs all day, wishing I was home. So I tried working from home, but blinding pain is immensely distracting. Both of these approaches taught me something key: If you are in mega pain, give your body and brain the rest they're asking for. Ice packs, heating pads, naps, meditation, acetaminophen, naproxen, ibuprofen... watch TV and disappear into a funny/dramatic/thoughtful world. Still keep trying to take a few steps and do not give up hope.

You have a "bad back" that may need a bit more TLC at times. You must be prepared to nurse it back to health. Don't forget that people "throw their backs out" all the time, scoliosis or not.[41] You're just used to more pain and your nervous system may be on higher alert. You are also likely more fed up with it, which will do nothing to calm down this kind of episode. Pain is exhausting.

Some days you may want a cane or walker to assist your pained gait. Leaning forward may be the only position where you can escape the pain. Lifting your feet to walk may be too much, so shuffling sounds like a great option. But odds are you *don't* need a walker since this episode shall pass. You are stronger than you think (even though you may not remember that too easily on those days). Take it easy, stretch gently the way your PSSE recommends, don't live entirely on the couch, rest when you need to, and keep putting one foot in front of the other.

These hips lie

At this point in the game, you have likely realized just how bendy your body can be. If you haven't, just look at how bendy your spine is (scoliosis humor). While there is solid structure to the body, we are not made entirely of bricks and mortar. This is really good news for a number of reasons. On a day-to-day basis, though, it can drive you a bit bananas.

Some days our bodies are completely off-center, skewed to one side, looking particularly asymmetrical and rotated. One wrist may rest against the hip bone, shoulders slanting, clothes falling lopsided; you may never guess that those particularly twisted days are sometimes pain-free! Your body has a pattern it *likes*, after all. And yet sometimes you're that askew and in *fantastic* pain.

Of course, there's the flipside too: the days when you appear perfectly symmetrical. Hips are aligned, nothing looks visibly out of whack, your clothes fall flawlessly... but *holy moly* is there screaming pain in there. And yet sometimes you're well aligned *and* pain-free. How annoying.

Adjust as needed for alignment, pain, and wardrobe, but your flexible body sometimes does what it wants.

PMS: pretty mighty scoliosis

Buckle up, ladies. It's about to get bad. That time of the month is fast approaching. You're all too familiar with PMS coming your way: the moods, the cramps, the crying at sad movies, the cramps, the feminine hygiene supplies box, the significant other steering clear for a few days, the cramps! It's so rough. Thank goodness men sympathize with us, but they really have no clue how bad it can be. Just a few days and you'll be in the clear...

Oh, wait! Silly me, I forgot about the *other* PMS that kicks in: pretty mighty scoliosis! That monthly dose of extra lower back pain that, combined with your uterus pain, makes your entire midsection one ginormous *ow* zone. Front and back. Double-sided.

We are all different, but if you're treated to the double PMS experience, you know this part just sucks. It is as hard to explain the feeling as it is to identify the source of the pain. We find ourselves wondering, "Is it PMS hurting my back or scoliosis? Do I need chocolate or a stretch?" (Probably both.) There's no escaping it, and you just have to wait it out. It might be some small comfort to know that you're not the only one. Let's support each other as we sandwich ourselves in between a heating pad and a hot water bottle… a PMS sandwich!

If you don't get to experience this, be very glad.

Bad moods courtesy of pain

Going to sleep in pain. Being awoken in the middle of the night by pain. Waking up in the morning in pain… Was it all a dream where somebody was trying to extract top-secret information out of me?

Oh wait… no, it's just my muscles and joints and who-knows-what-else having a flare-up, mad about the activity I did (or lack of). Nothing to be (too) concerned with… No top-secret information here… No immediate end to this torture. It's enough to drive a person mad after a while.

Apparently when the pain doesn't give you a minute's break in 24-plus hours, your *mood* can change. In the notes of my first scoliosis appointment, the doctor wrote down that I was "a pleasant young lady." Fast forward a couple years and that had gone right out the window. Pain pain pain can *zap* good moods right out of you.

I once spent an afternoon paddleboarding with my best friend at my uncle's lakeside cottage, blissfully enjoying a Canadian summer day. I could feel my back straining with every stroke of the paddle. Wouldn't you know, the next morning I could barely stand up. My saintly friend had to physically pull me up out of bed to standing using our foolproof system we call "The Morning Haul." But she could only do so much, and I had to *slowly, painstakingly* make my way to the breakfast table.

It was raining, I felt like I was 200 years old, and I was ready to pack it in and go home. In fact, I was so exhausted from the pain alone that I took two long naps that day. I was completely wiped out. By the evening, I needed to resort to a couple of prescription pain pills for the night. I slept intermittently for a few more hours and woke up less than enthused to a perfect sunny day greeting me. "That's it," I told myself. "Enough is enough. You're going to do something about this *now* because you have two more gorgeous days at this lake and you're not going to be in a pained *bad mood* for it." I threw on some walking clothes and headed towards the main road, determined to get some fresh air and do motion therapy instead of lying down and letting that bad mood grow.

Well, the great Canadian bugs had other plans. The July mosquitoes swarmed me instantly on the paved road and I was forced to beat a hasty retreat back to the cabin. Onto Plan B: "Dear Uncle, is there anything – *anything* – that needs to be done around here? I cannot sit still or sleep away another full day. I am so *sore* and *grumpy*. Any light manual labor I could do? Do you need firewood by the campfire? Is there a path that needs cleaning? Lawns that need mowing?"

As a normal human, my uncle was baffled by this request from somebody with a "bad back." Wouldn't I rather lie down on the floor? But he found us an overgrown area of brush that he wanted cleaned up, and off to work we went! Within 20 minutes, I was walking normally again, my hips loose and my muscles unlocked. He pulled me aside and said, "I just can't believe how much better you look just from moving around and doing some work. I didn't know how to help, but this is honestly the last thing I would have offered you." My immediate reply to him is what shocked me the most out of this whole story, causing me to stop and think about it afterwards: "I'm a joyful person when I'm not in pain."

I realized right there just how much pain can take over, right down to your mood. Pain was often the last thing I felt when falling asleep and the first thing I felt when waking up. An entire day's activities could be based on how much *ow* was present. A whole day's schedule could go right out the window if it was really bad, especially in the lower back.

The trick is to be the one in control, knowing what you need to do to care for that pain and your resulting mood – don't let it zap your joy. It can take time to find the combo that works for you. Part of it, as I've heard from too many scolis, is the frustration involved in discovering your own personal blend of solutions – there is no one-size-fits-all how-to-handle-your-scoliosis-without-a-doubt manual to give you and send you on your way. Take the time to stop and see how you can address your pain, take note of it, and build upon your own manual. Might I suggest you include in it a hot shower to course over those pained zones.

Note: I have only experienced paddleboarding as a fusioneer. Some warriors with different backs *love* paddleboarding. For me it is quite hard on the lower back, whether I am sitting or standing. Maybe there are adjustments that could be made that I haven't been clued in to yet. If it's not working out for you, why not try another water sport, like kayaking with a built-in back support?

Paingry

Have you ever been "hangry"? You know, when you're so hungry you become angry? How about "paingry"? When you're in so much pain you simply cannot endure *it* or *yourself* anymore and become agitated? It's the next level past "bad moods." I am not at liberty to say which is more dangerous between "hangry" or "paingry." But what I can say with confidence is that hangry has a quick fix, while paingry has no guarantee of rapid resolution.

Painger can be frustrating, to say the least. You cannot simply devour a granola bar and be "safe" for a little while. If seated, you may get up and try to walk a few circles to shake it off. If already standing, you may grab a seat on the closest edge available, even if it's a sidewalk curb. You begin to desperately seek anything to shift your body's weight into a new direction, hoping against hope that it will alleviate some pain. This seems like it should be feasible. The trouble is, if you're already at the "paingry" state, your pain has built up past the "mild discomfort" stage well into the "I am going to *end* somebody if I don't get an ounce of relief soon" stage. Did you hear the angry part of pain in there?

Painger frustration is rare, thankfully, but very real. (If you are a scoli with little to no pain, you are wondrously lucky and are unlikely to experience painger. Take it as a win.) Painger is not something that other museum visitors want to witness; nor are paingry emotions something you want showing through when you're in mid-presentation at school or work. The best I can recommend is to carry snacks with you to stave off any hanger – you don't want a double whammy of hanger-painger.

Painsomnia

This one is apt to ruin your tonight and your tomorrow. There's no timing it or taking any educated guess as to when or if it might happen. You only find out once it's too late… literally.

I never had any sleep troubles before high school. In fact, pre-scoliosis, I never woke up at night, rarely had nightmares, and was always the early bird. By my junior year, constant pain had fully settled in, paired with the fear of the unknown and surgery. It's all too easy for your mind to get hung up on those big life topics and let them run around in your head in circles, particularly at the end of the day when you're finally alone with your own thoughts. I wasn't completely alone though: I also had my night brace. All were catalysts for sleepless nights. The devil on my shoulder wanted to rip open the brace to get comfier, but the angel on the other side would warn me that every night spent in the brace could help counter the bends. *Arghhh!* How can any teenager sleep with such a pandemonium of life decisions and worry bashing around in their brain, while in *pain*?

As a foolish teenager, I didn't tell anybody about my sleep problems. By the time my quality sleep had dwindled to a handful of hours most nights, I was so grumpy during the day that my classmates chalked it up to a personality trait. Not sleeping well takes its toll on anybody. The less sleep I got, the lower my pain tolerance was. The more pain I felt, the more frustrated I became. The madder I became, the more worries I had about a future like this with or without surgery. These were also the years I discovered makeup, particularly concealer, which I applied liberally to hide my nighttime ruminating.

After surgery, my sleeping improved substantially. With that big scary decision-hurdle over and done with, I felt like I could get on with my life and handle whatever came my way. This lasted for quite a number of years, until – lo and behold – my back pain began to act up again. Being sore and uncomfortable became the new catalyst for dropping me right back into old habits of worrying about the future and getting mad at the pain.

Over the years, truly learning about my spine and scoliosis empowered me to silence many of those worries. Now the handful of short nights I experience have me thinking about pain progression, what I should or could be doing to improve my health overall for a better quality of life, how genetic scoliosis *really* is, and how best to work an eight-hour desk job every day for the next 30 years... the same fear of unknowns, but now with an inquisitive lens rather than a scared or angry one.

It is still good general self-care to create the best sleep environment possible. Do all you can to boost your sleep! Anything that favors serotonin should be given a chance.[42] Charge all devices outside of the bedroom and refuse to look at them past a certain time. Get as much fresh air and exercise as possible throughout the day, and go for a relaxed walk around the block for a dose of fresh air and movement before bed. Stretch before bed to release the tightness that built up over the day. Watch or read something you find enjoyable and light, avoiding news, violence, or sad content in the evening.

Once in bed, do your prayers or some breathing exercises, focusing on where the air is flowing through your body – tuning in can calm other rampant thoughts while grounding you in the moment.

Melatonin pills are available over the counter, but your body knows how to produce that itself. Liquid sleep aids are available too, but you can develop a tolerance to them, which can lead to needing to guzzle more and more of it over time.[43] Speak with your doctor if you have trouble sleeping and find out what best options are available for *you*. They can direct you to counseling of some sort, recommend fresh air and exercise (my default self-prescription in adulthood), and maybe some medical sleep aids.

In the meantime, there's a big world of serotonin-inducing activities and joy out there. Find what makes you *happy*!

Days with zero pain

For anybody who has weekly pains, these no-pain days just seem brighter! Anything seems possible. You find yourself well-rested, bouncing around and dancing down hallways. You move with fluidity and can do whatever you like without an "*ow*."

Revel in it. Don't start questioning the "whys" or "hows." You know how they say, "Enjoy the little things in life"? Well, this is one of those little things for us.

MUST GET PHYSICAL

Motion is lotion

Hear me out! Moving, jumping, running, using your *whole* body... it's all hearty stuff! Wake up those sleepy muscles that are used to being cemented in a scoliosis formation. Thaw out those sections frozen in place around a fusion. Give a break to the overworked muscles that spend every moment holding you up. Try it out and you might discover a physical therapy that's fun, sociable, and affordable! Throughout each week, aim to do some mix of the following: stretching, strength training, cardio, balance training, and something outdoors. Some of us have come to view "going to the gym" as "going to the spa" – we feel so good when we walk out of there. It can also be easier to stay motivated when it's about your *health* and not just your *appearance*.

If you're already active and sporty, that's great! Keep it up! If you're not, then build up some courage and try out some activities. There are tons of scolis out there running, lifting weights, cycling, rock climbing, dancing... It might take some time to find the right one for you, but along the way, you're sure to meet new people and have new experiences – variety is the spice of life! Keep in mind that it's generally easier to be motivated when you work out in a group rather than forcing yourself to move on your own. It is also an automatic morale booster and builds confidence since we are social creatures (even though our health can easily make us want to retreat into solitude).

The stereotypical "scoliosis sports" that are immediately suggested for strengthening and pain relief are yoga and swimming. Give them a try if you haven't already – many warriors live by some combination of yoga, Pilates, and swimming. However, I'll admit I left more than one class midway through in frustrated tears because my back was in pain or I was unable to follow along with the bending or rotation demands. A fairly recent development is scoli- and fusion-friendly yoga and Pilates classes, which can kick those frustrations of "I can't do it because of my fusion" or "every spine in here can do this except mine" to the curb. These activities are also fantastic for re-training your breath

Turns out we can still do just about anything post-op! But it may take some time and adjustments.

If you're a dancer, it will slowly come back to you as your body heals. You may need to learn new ways of moving, but it hasn't stopped *many* fused dancers from continuing with it for years and years. The community's advice is to steer clear of backbends, though, including the party game "Limbo." Running comes back too – you just need to relearn to walk before you can run.

Soccer, basketball, volleyball, hiking, biking... it's all still there for you to do. Maybe you can even work your way up to a sports scholarship! A fellow fusioneer competes in rock climbing at the summer Olympics. Winter Olympic sports like skiing and skating are also up for grabs. Snowboarding has been reported as trickier and sometimes simply not possible, since a large component of it is holding yourself in a spinal rotation. I can attest that sitting on the snowy ground and reaching for snowboard bindings without the ability to arch forward can be incredibly frustrating.

Beach volleyball became my go-to team sport. During one game, I had to tuck down to cover my face when a wild ball came at me from another court. Crouched down with my arms folded over my head and my back flatly open to missiles, that volleyball bounced right into the center of my scar. I flattened out onto the sand on impact, my brain going into auto-scan mode to make sure everything was okay and my rods were not upset. Of course, I was totally fine from a pleather ball hitting me. My friends were by my side in a millisecond since I was a little spooked. Nothing like that had yet happened to me post-op! I got up, dusted off the sand, walked off the court, and took a water break with a guy in the group I had never met before – a friend of a friend in town for the weekend. Naturally, we got to talking about the scene that just took place. He kicked it off with, "I have a really bad back, and I felt it when I saw you drop down. I have something called scoliosis. Not many people really know what it is." Well didn't I just stop dead in my tracks. I had to catch my breath to reply, "Ya, I know *exactly* what that is. I had surgery for it a couple years ago and that's why I dropped like a rock when it hit me!" We had a wonderful water break together as I comfortably chatted about scoliosis with a stranger for the first time in my life.

There are scolis and fusioneers out there doing all kinds of sports, likely with adjustments. Scolis are not always built for all "standard" exercises, so we need to draft our own workout handbooks – learn how to work out for *yourself*, not for anybody else and not necessarily in the same way they do. Don't worry about looking different than the other participants. It's about how you *feel* during and after. The most important rule when exercising: Don't push it if it hurts. If your body is telling you it doesn't like something, even if everybody else is doing it, listen to your body *first*.

Always check with your doctors before trying anything big and new after surgery to make sure you're cleared for it. You can still get a great workout or stretch – just talk with your PSSE therapist, who can recommend how to adjust the exercise specifically for you.[44]

Going for walks

As I sit at my desk writing this section, I can feel a deep desire to go for a walk. It's like there's a happy golden retriever deep inside my soul, wagging her tail and looking up expectantly, "Walk? We go for walk? Outside? Yeah, yeah, yeah! Walk!"

Moving your body is your second business, part-time job, side hustle, whatever you want to call it. It may be time out of your day, but it is time well spent *not* sitting! Enjoy an opportunity to *not sit* and also gain an appreciation that you are *able* to move. It doesn't have to be anything extreme. Super long walks can cause other pains, as reported by fellow scolis. Take the dog for a walk or ask the neighbor if you can borrow their dog. Use TV commercial breaks to go get something from another room. Get off the bus a stop or two early when going to work and walk those extra blocks instead. Join your coworkers for a walk to the coffee shop, even if you're not going to buy anything. Walk to a restaurant instead of taking a cab.

Gently loosen that lower back and hip zone after a length of time sitting in a forced 90-degree fold of tightness in the front. Alternate different parts of the spine that are taking on the load with each step.[45] Get the blood pumping through all the muscles that work so hard for you around the clock, moving your weight around and engaging different pieces. Oh, and those shoulders, confined to typing at a keyboard, neck forward to stare into a computer monitor, straining despite the best ergonomic setup available. Let's get those arms moving naturally once again! Maybe a mini backbend midway through the stroll. Notice how strong you are and thank yourself for taking the time to care for *you*.

Yet another gift from this activity? After you've been standing for a while, you get to sit back down again! *Ahhhh.* How good does that feel? Taking the weight off the soles of your feet, changing formation again, getting back into a seated state.

There are 24 hours in a day; surely you can carve out some time to go outside and treat yourself to some free movement therapy.

Engage your core

It took me years to figure out what a "core" was, what it felt like, and how to engage those muscles. The fitness instructors who said, "Tuck in your belly," apparently already knew what a "core" was and seemingly couldn't explain it any other way. Meanwhile, some of us have never engaged those muscles in a sit-up before in our *life*. What the heck does "engage your core" actually mean?

It's *not* sucking in your gut, taking a big breath of air into your lungs, or trying to look super slim at the belly. In my experience, it's substantially tougher to instantly engage your core when it feels like you have little or no core to engage. If you find yourself frustrated with this concept, know you're not the only one. Take it easy on yourself if you don't understand what the pros are talking about yet.

There are a lot of "beginner ab workouts" online but be wary which you pick. Some may be easier to engage your back muscles instead. Others might be fast-paced and leave room for error or injury. Most don't consider scoli implications. Don't forget that your body is a little bit different from the "general" body those workouts were designed for.

To make sure you're learning key exercises properly, consider visiting a certified pro like an instructor of *scoliosis*-specific yoga, Pilates, strengthening, or PSSE therapist to get you started with modified core exercises for *your* back. I hurt myself more than once doing sit-ups like everybody else or yoga poses that were modified for me (with good intentions) by a yoga instructor who *didn't* understand scoliosis. There's nothing quite like a personalized education, especially for an investment that will serve you for the rest of your life without angering your scoliosis. A little bit of correct information can go a long way!

It's important to keep in mind that nothing – including fitness – happens overnight. You don't need to start at the Olympic level because you are likely *not* an Olympian. You are just trying to start somewhere and get better. And it *will* get better as long as you put in the effort.

Counter-stretching. All. The. Time.

Wake-up time. Stretch. Break time. Stretch. Lunch time. Stretch. Quitting time. Stretch. Traffic time. Stretch. Dinner time. Stretch. Midnight snack time. Stretch. Sleepy time… Zzz… Repeat.

It feels like your delinquent muscles want to go left, but your obedient muscles want to go right. Get those props: roll on the exercise balls, stretch out with the elastics, hit the mat for deep stretches, get into a neutral position with the wedges, reach for the sky and breathe. You need to appease your body and mind that keep saying *ow* somehow. It's so easy to become a rinse-and-repeat routine, though, and quite honestly it can get tiresome. Your personal back maintenance can become an annoying part-time job.

Negativity can easily creep in. "Think of all the things you could do," it says, "if you didn't have to spend so much time stretching, counter-curving, and counter-rotating yourself. You could be making money, seeing friends, stopping to smell the roses. You wouldn't have to plan stretch breaks into your day and could get more office work done to impress the boss." Sure, tiny devil voice, that's not necessarily incorrect, but where will that thinking get us? Nowhere fast. Instead, train the bouncy little positive voice to pipe up. "Yeah, this is taking up some of your time," it trills, "but is it really all that bad? Every cat and dog wakes up with a great *big* stretch… every day of its life. Let's keep stretching to limber up throughout the day. And let's keep learning about our body and nervous system!"

Your nervous system, by the way, consists of your brain, spinal cord, and a matrix of nerves throughout your entire body; together they relay all kinds of messages between your brain and body.[46] Everything is able to work together through this system – eyes, ears, heart, lungs, automatic and voluntary movements…. Some nervous systems that live in a state of stress become quite sensitive and slow to calm down; other people's nervous systems are quite relaxed.[47] Understanding the complexities of the nervous system can help you better understand scoliosis side-effects. It's a good topic to learn more about on your own time, especially if you're in pain or finding the benefits of stretching aren't lasting.

Whatever you choose to do, be sure your stretches are right for *your* unique back. Sometimes what feels good to your mind does not actually advance your own best interests and alignment. Be sure to check in with a scoliosis-trained therapist every now and then to identify stretches best for *you*. Bodies can change; they benefit from regular check-ups.

Becoming an expert in your treatments

Just a reminder that we live in the modern era with tons of treatment options available to us. Bracing, surgery, and "wait and see" are not always the "only way forward"; there are other options and combos depending on the situation. Be aware that many people benefit from some physical therapy, but many types of therapy can become short-term solutions to alleviate pain without addressing the core problem. It's important to not just chase constant pain relief but, rather, learn about and strengthen the *right* muscles for *your* body. You have to actively put in the work too.

It can be intimidating to set out on a physical therapy quest. "Where do I start? What do I need? My other healthcare professionals haven't provided me with many options or advice." Over time, it may even become discouraging – you've consulted numerous practitioners, and nobody's been able to *really* help you with their methods. You've picked up some good stretches or techniques here and there, learning about the human body, but the alignment and pain still isn't being addressed... Don't worry, you're not alone.

Step 1: Find a human who can teach you about your unique scoliosis back and all of the moving pieces around it, not just some general-purpose guide online. Bring your X-rays to a physical therapist who knows *a lot* about scoliosis and orthopaedics. Consider training one-on-one with a professional scoli-yoga or scoli-Pilates teacher.

Unfortunately, many medical teams don't clue scolis in to the existence of scoliosis-specific exercises. Some warriors spend years traveling across their country seeking out general-purpose therapists (who don't fully understand the intricacies of scoliosis) in the hopes they will remove their pain, but ultimately they have little to no effect. After over a decade of trying out chiro after physio after physio after massage after sports medicine after painful physio after kinesiologist after massage after acupuncture after physio (that list could go on for a while), I finally discovered scoli-specific physiotherapy. Walking into that treatment room was the *first* time I felt like I was in the right place: The walls were covered in pictures of spines and backs that looked *just like mine*. For the first time in my entire painful saga, I was not confronted with "straight-spine" pictures that made me feel different and I was not left trying to imagine what my back was actually doing while receiving treatment – I could see it right in front of me.

My quest for "physical therapy that actually works" led to another crashing realization once I was finally in that PSSE office, where I was assessed and treated while in a sports bra. I actually got in a bit of trouble for wearing a sports bra that covered my back *too much*. Why is this significant? Because it was the first time any physical therapist actually wanted to *see* my spine, muscles, and structures, and how they were all working together. Hindsight being 20/20, why had no other therapist been interested in what my back and scoliosis were doing while they were giving me handfuls of exercises? Previously I always wore t-shirts or thin sweaters while being assessed, painfully treated, or exercised. It is impossible to see what is truly going on under a sweater!

Step 2: Learn as much as you can about *your* back and the effect scoliosis has had on it. It helps knowing what your specific structure is as you start working with it since you kind of become your own body builder.

You can't begin to help your own body daily if you know nothing about it – you need to know what you're dealing with! I learned more about my own special scoli back in *one* session of Schroth than in all of those years of general-purpose back specialists *combined*. Just a few months into Schroth, I already noticed a difference in how my body was responding to breath and movement. By tuning in to my body and following expert guidance, I finally began breathing into my concavities (and finally clued in to the fact I had "concavities," among other key scoli-structures). At last, there was hope! It was immensely empowering to learn about *my* alignment and breath, and direct how it *should* work instead of being subjected to how it *wants* to work. I was finally in command. That's it, body... No more running rampant and moving however you feel like. No more trying to figure it all out from a scoli-free back on the internet that isn't *yours*. And certainly no more "innocently" incorrect information from non-scoliosis back professionals. Not only that, my new expert finally explained the recurring pains I'd lived with *for over a decade* and painful instances where I "threw out my back." This is an education on how to best care for your scoli back *for life*.

Step 3: Do the exercises! Scoli-specific exercises involve stabilizing and breathing into specific areas to strengthen and elongate. Of course, nothing worth having is ever easy.

These exercises can be tough, awkward, and sometimes uncomfortable. Tears may happen with any physical therapy exercises – it can be frustrating trying to make your body change how it wants to hang out. But if these exercises were super easy, fun, and fancy-free, they probably wouldn't be providing any benefit and change. Like all exercises, give it your best shot.

At the beginning, you may want to take a lot of notes and pictures to refer to as you practice your exercises to make sure you're doing them right. That's more than okay. As you become more familiar with the exercises and your muscles get the hang of them, you'll need to refer to those notes and pictures less and less. If you find yourself getting frustrated, just take a pause and come back to the exercises later in the day... but never give up. Take it one day at a time, and remember that any small progress is still progress.

Looking back, I can't fathom doing the reverse order: going from scoliosis-specific treatments to generic treatments. A large gap of information would have presented itself immediately. Instead, that information gap took me years to identify and fill – here's hoping my story will help you on your physical therapy search.

A caution: Be wary of specialists who oversell their "solutions" and get you hooked on their services. Businesses may broadly claim they can help with all "back pain"... Be sure to ask about scoliosis specifically. I've heard "Yes, of course! We do it all!" too many times with absolutely no relief or results. Be extra cautious of physical therapists who claim they can magically "cure" scoliosis – there is no total cure. You may even move from one therapist to another, who immediately says, "Oh, of course your last one didn't work for you. It's not as good as what we do *here*! *We* can help you." Different professionals don't always see eye-to-eye either. It's a fine balance of trusting the experts but also knowing your own body. Do your own research into the data. What kind of results has their type of therapy shown over the years? Evidence-based research will save you time and energy.

On that note, *each and every body is different*. Some scolis don't do any physical therapy other than the occasional massage to release muscle tightness from naughty, knotty scoliosis. Others love a dose of myofascial release at home each morning (which a myofascial physiotherapist can teach you about). Some non-fusioneers like chiropractic adjustments here and there; others absolutely refuse it. Even if you have a fusion, there are still many moving parts around it that could likely use some PSSE guidance. It all comes down to what *you* are looking for and what *you* can realistically commit to.

And now a couple of firsthand experiences to share...

While fusion recovery doesn't always mandate physical therapy, I was told to give it a try if I wanted to. So... with no further guidance provided by the hospital, I gave it a try! But I chose poorly. I visited a sports medicine physio, who hooked me up to a TENS machine ("TENS" stands for transcutaneous electrical nerve stimulation). It's a little electrical box with wires strategically hooked up around your pained area that sends low-voltage currents through you to provide pain relief.[48] Let me tell you in no unclear terms: Do not opt into this *around your scar* mere months after your surgery. Your incision will still be tender, and that area has been through enough. My experience left me sobbing, hooked up to a zap box around my healing incision while the sports physio went off to check on another client in the open-area treatment zone. TENS certainly helps some folks with pain pre-op, or post-op in areas *other* than the incision. There are even at-home kits you can keep around.

Then there was the time I gave the mesmerizing world of acupuncture a whirl. This has potential with some acupuncturists and less so with others. A lot of people have basic training in acupuncture,[49] but to reap the full benefits it can offer, it's really best to go with a pro. Somebody who does this almost exclusively will know every pinpoint of release available and be able to better target your unique spine. Once again, try finding one who knows about scoliosis! I visited one lady who claimed to be able to help, but once she saw my pre-op back in the nude she exclaimed, "Ohhh, *woahhh*. What's that?" Not exactly what you want to hear from somebody who is about to turn you into a pincushion. Make sure to check out their qualifications and reviews beforehand.

Let's not forget a key area mentioned throughout these pages: emotional health. Scoliosis affects more than just the physical body that practitioners can knead and that you can help align at home; there is a psychological side to scoliosis. Emotional support and education are also very important. Remember, it's all connected! Just like with physical therapists, it can take time to find a psychological therapist who can support your scoliosis journey.

You may have already found some therapist or some therapy that works wonders for you. That's great! If you're still searching the market for something that fits your needs, don't give up. It can be overwhelming to figure out where to start and what to do, and frustrating when you need to reinitiate the search. Take a look online, read reviews, and ask people around you for recommendations. Scoliosis is unique to every patient; you should have a custom explanation and set of exercises *just for you*. Invest in this education for yourself. Do the corrective exercises to tackle that feeling of asymmetry and relieve discomfort for the long run. You may be freshly done with bracing and surgery, and want to take a total break from all treatments and exercises, but don't stop caring for yourself or your back. You have made great progress and need to keep it up. It's all a part of the TLC dance with scoliosis.

Note: Non-scoli people often have no idea how much time, energy, effort, money, and frustration goes into your physical therapy. After all, you're not a pro right away and figuring out all these exercises takes time and patience. Not to mention you're pushing your body against itself (kind of) to make these exercises work. You're not "just" lying on the floor or sitting on a chair; you're totally tuned in, vigilantly watching for any overcompensations and focusing your breath into specific areas. *Phew!* That's a lot of effort.

Additional note: Perhaps the worst feeling in doctor/patient interactions is when you, the patient, are made to feel *absolutely* irresponsible for wanting to try out a different treatment option. You may have discovered something new through your own research, or maybe a fellow scoli recommended what worked well for them. When a scoliosis treatment doesn't fall under your doctor's list of "legitimate" treatments, they may physically look *down* at you as they tell you why even considering it is foolish. Being made to feel terrible as you search for solutions feels… terrible.

CONSIDERATIONS

Gravity

The unrelenting force of gravity is weighing down on you at every moment. Thankfully (thankfully!) we don't feel its full effect. We just amble on with our daily lives, blissfully grounded to the surface of the Earth without floating away uncontrollably. This is a very good thing. However, some days there is just so much compression in your spine that you start thinking if somebody would just FOR THE LOVE OF ALL THAT IS GOOD TURN DOWN THE GRAVITY, then your spine would extend a bit on its own for some sweet respite.

Just a bit. Just for a couple of minutes. It's cranked up way too high. You feel squished in all the wrong spots. You just want to give your organs some room to breathe. One hip and rib cage are about to touch; one shoulder is higher than the other and the neck is compensating for it. Give us a break from the forces pushing down on our coiled vertebrae. The worst is that, thanks to said scoliosis and/or fusion, it can feel next to impossible to stretch it all out. Instead, we often feel irked at the shape we're forced into.

Since changing the forces of the cosmos may be too much of an ask, it's a good thing humans continue to use their giant brains to invent tools to *counter* gravity. Zero gravity chair, anybody? Yes, *please*! Although you cannot spend every minute of every day in one of these brilliant inventions, there's nothing stopping you from popping into one now and then. No shame in playing the anti-gravity game.

Money talks

Deep tissue massage, physiotherapy, chiropractor, acupuncture, myofascial, PSSE, fitness classes, pool access, personal trainers, clothing, equipment, props, braces, hospitals, surgery, medicine… it can add up quickly.

When you're first tackling this curvature as well as any pain, you may not have experience in all the types of treatments available. It's not your fault – you're new to this! Keep in mind the long-term results you are seeking (versus actually receiving) as you balance your budget.

In the movie of *My Spine*, I cast many a physical therapist in lead roles, but in the end *spoiler alert* I discovered I was the main character! All of those casting calls added up to thousands of dollars and countless hours paying over and over again for what turned out to be temporary pain relief. Once I understood which offered temporary pain relief and which actually addressed my scoli structure, it went from a star-studded over-budget Hollywood production with no meat to an indie film that really hit home.

Aside from treatment, the bracing and hospital costs can give the fitness bills a run for their money. A back brace costs *thousands* of dollars – and some children need multiple braces as they grow. If the curves progress to require surgery, you're looking at surgery, hospital room, parking, and medication fees – none of which are cheap.

The final cost of overall therapy, bracing, and surgery is also largely affected by where you live and work. Sometimes there is subsidized healthcare, private healthcare, or insurance benefits through work. Sometimes costs fall to the patient to figure out. Thankfully there are resources to help with the financial side of scoliosis. Look for foundations and charities in your country that offer aid for bracing, medication, hospital, transportation, or lodging costs.

Music

Feeling frustrated? Boogie down! Feeling tight in the hips? Dance it out! Furious from twinges and pains around your spine? Rock on!

More than ever, music is at our fingertips. We don't have to scan the radio to find something that moves us; nor do we have to go down to a brick-and-mortar store to buy a CD that we may or may not like. We have dozens of streaming options available online! You can cruise through unlimited songs, artists, and genres until you find something that releases your frustration and/or sore muscles. Build yourself a little "mood boost" playlist with all of your faves!

Some hospitals have music therapists included as part of the surgical recovery team. They come by to sing and play instruments for (or with) patients. Some fusioneers who could only sit a few minutes at a time alone in their recovery room found that music therapy allowed them to sit up for an hour completely at ease!

There have been countless studies done correlating music with healing.[50] Even if you're not musically inclined, you just need to listen to something that speaks to you and your brain takes it in as medicine.

Scoliosis fashion

Just because scoliosis pops up in your life, your personal fashion style does not have to change. Allow me to be very clear about this: You can *totally* wear what you want! Do not let scoliosis stop you from being you and expressing yourself.

Just like everybody else buying clothes to flatter their body types, scoliosis may just shift your choices towards fits that compliment your body. It may direct you to select certain cuts and types of fabric over others. Remember that not every article of clothing is meant to fit every body anyway! Good thing we have racks upon racks of items and designs to choose from. Some neck lines may sit funny on one shoulder. Some waistlines may sit on a higher hip resulting in one shorter pant leg. Some warriors avoid striped shirts and tight tops. Others avoid belts at the waist and don't tuck their blouses into their pants since these accentuate their curves.

Bracers love sweaters that are easy to toss on in the winter and breathable fabrics for the summer. It could be way trickier – baggy shirts and sweaters are *super* comfy and completely acceptable in today's world. If this were the 1950s, when ladies wore heels and dresses, it would be another story altogether… A moment of silence for our ladies from the '50s. How on earth did they manage without modern medicine and baggy sweaters?

Wear what makes *you* feel good.

A back is just a back. It's a body part that can be bared in public without any legal problems, if you wish. Just like an arm or leg, you can choose to show it off or keep it warm and covered. If there's a scar, you can apply sunscreen and let it breathe, or use a shirt to protect it from the sun's rays. *It's your choice.*

If you haven't shown the world any part of your back in a while, you can feel ever so naked the first time you expose it. You could be wearing a string bikini with a *cape* and feel more decent than uncovering your pale back to the wind! Remember… it's okay. It's your body, and you get to choose how much you want to reveal or cover up – that's true even if you *don't* have scoliosis. Once again, every body is different, and everybody is different. Some want to display a scar right away in all its glory; others want to take some time getting to know it first before showing the world. Both are okay! (Did I mention? It's your choice.)

I was always comfortable in a bikini around my familiar people, but it took a while to do so around strangers. Pre-surgery, I would buy bikinis that tied up in the back with a big bow to fill-in my concavity. Post-fusion, I prefer ones that tie up in the front and are flat around the back to avoid the pressure of a knot on my incision when I'm sitting in a beach chair or lying on the sand. That's the personal preference of *one* scoli in a bikini (me); you should rock whatever style you like! (All together now... It's your choice!)

In the realm of bras, ladies, you are not the only one constantly having to tighten one strap more than the other because of your bends. Nor are you the only one forever repositioning bra straps that insist on sliding off one shoulder.

I have spoken to so many gorgeous bracers, fusioneers, and natural scolis who pay *zero* mind to their braces, scars, and prominences. After all, they're just a part of our life story and there's nothing to hide. Many have been empowered by other warriors posting open-back support pictures online – how wonderful is our community! No matter what you choose to wear or to show or not show, dress in what makes *you* feel comfortable and safe. For some of us, open-back dresses and bikinis may not be on that list. Surround yourself with a loving support system of people who care about *you* and not about what you wear.

Remember that you are your own customer, so you do *you*, whatever that may be! If you have a fusion, you also know the challenge of rotating your torso to see how the back of your outfit looks. Thank goodness there are mirrors to help us out!

Need some inspiration?

Seeking a boost in your scoliosis world today? Scoli celebrities can swoop in to make us feel better. As with every scoliosis case, every scoli celebrity is different. Some are in pain; others have no pain. Some have had bracing and avoided surgery; others did not have success with bracing. Some have a thoracic curve, a lumbar curve, or both. Some play golf, while others will not. But the one thing they all have in common is this: Scoliosis has not held them back from being successful and attaining their dreams. You can find their stories online.

Let's start with the movies! Alongside Sarah Michelle Gellar, there's the classic Elizabeth Taylor, Liza Minnelli, Rene Russo, Vanessa Williams, Laura

Dern, Chloë Sevigny, Shailene Woodley, Rita Simons, Isabella Rossellini and her daughter Elettra Wiedemann, and many more.

Scoli models include Ayesha Jones, Rebecca Romijn, and Martha Hunt. Scoli singers include Anne Murray, Jessica Andrews, Melanie Blatt, and Kurt Cobain. Elsewhere in the entertainment industry, there's comedian Carmen Lynch, news host Giuliana Rancic, Miss North Carolina Katherine Southard, and famed cellist Yo-Yo Ma.

Sports more your style? There's no shortage of determination, motivation, and resilience in these athletes! Jeanette Lee is a professional pool player who's had 10 surgeries on her back and neck. There are many scoli swimmers like Maritza Correia, Jessica Ashwood, and David Popovici. How about pro golfer Stacy Lewis, Olympic climber Kyra Condie, tennis champ James Blake, and Olympic sprinter Usain Bolt? There are powerlifters, football players, dancers… all kinds of athletes who are curved and continue to make the most of their goals!

A fan of royalty? Princess Eugenie of the British Royal family had spinal fusion for her scoliosis at age 12. She has spoken quite openly about it and wore a wedding dress that purposely displayed her upper scar. Let's throw it back a bit further to King Richard III of England, who was thought to have a hunch (according to Shakespeare). When they unearthed his bones in 2012, however, they discovered he had a curve ranging from 70 to 90 degrees.[51]

Did you know that US General Douglas MacArthur had scoliosis? He was denied entry into West Point Academy because of it, deemed "medically unfit" even though he aced all of his other tests. He found a doctor who would work with him, did his prescribed exercises for a full year, went back to West Point, and was told that although he made great progress he was once again denied. He didn't give up, continuing with the exercises for a few more months and was finally accepted into the officer school.[52] How much determination and work did that require of him? A lot.

Incredible perseverance all around. Remind yourself that scoliosis does *not* have to be in your way. It may be a tough journey but something beautiful can come from it.

NOT DESIGNED WITH YOU IN MIND

Hammocks

No back support and completely at the mercy of a concave bag suspended by trees?

No thanks.

Hard chairs

Spinal curves and rotations can reveal themselves in areas next to the spine, especially in the thoracic area as rib prominences. When one rib cage is larger than the other, the more prominent side touches the back of any chair before the smaller side. That means the larger side rests against that uncomfortable chairback much longer. That can hurt after a while!

You can find yourself sitting there as long as you can endure, correcting your position as best you can, but eventually you keep sinking into the side with the dent – your concavity. Through all of this recorrecting, readjusting, and (essentially) squirming, your larger rib cage grinds against the chairback, never losing contact. Sit in any metal folding chair, wooden rocking chair, bar stool with a short backrest, or park bench for long enough, and you may very well walk away with a bruise branded across your prominent rib cage. *Ow.*

Footwear

Your feet are always doing something. Even if they're lying on the couch, they're still involved in pumping blood back up to your heart. They are the roots of your body and deserve to be treated well.

There are some strategic decisions to be made when it comes to footwear. It bears mentioning again: Every body is different. Some footwear fits better and others hurt more. Just like other clothing, you can wear any footwear that you *can* and *want* to wear. Some people have no problem throwing on $10 shoes with no arch support and walking for miles. Others love a thick heel. Many opt for "sensible footwear" with tight laces.

For those of us whose backs do *not* feel happy in stiletto heels, being pitched forward and messing with our balance, there's nothing forcing us to wear them.

Lower heels or thicker bases like wedges can feel much more solid and comfortable. (Just ask my feet – they spent years figuring that out the hard way.) We may still keep a couple pairs of fancy heels around for special occasions, or for when we're being driven door-to-door at primarily seated events, but we're not about to torture ourselves daily for something that doesn't work for us. Beauty may be pain, but if you're already in pain it's not worth it. You still look amazing!

Kitchens

Get dirty dishes, bend down, lean into the dishwasher to place them on the racks, stand up, and repeat and repeat and repeat. Heck, you'd wash them all by hand at this point if standing still at a sink looking down didn't hurt too! (Tip: Use a footstool to accompany sink duties to change your position or an anti-fatigue mat under your feet. Also applies to standing while cooking.)

Things you have to do about three times a day should not be difficult to reach. Dishwashers should load themselves. When is *that* technology arriving? My political campaign promise: Less bending for all with countertop dishwashers. Until then, everybody gets *one* standard-issue bowl and fork. My back can't handle the dishwasher today.

As for low-to-the-floor storage like those pesky deep corner cabinets... Realistically, what is supposed to be stored there? It'd better be something I need once a year, because there is no graceful arching low into that cupboard once there's a fusion. I will try to kneel and reach (to no avail), ultimately lying down on the floor in a prone position to snatch the item buried deep and low in the back corner. It simultaneously provides an excellent view of the corner moldings under the cabinet that are desperately in need of a good vacuuming. Excellent.

Working at the kitchen counter can be a pain... literally. You're standing immobile for a long time, your vertebrae are not taking on the load in the most efficient manner thanks to scoliosis, and you're looking straight down, pulling at your shoulders and the back of your neck. Should the need to cook for a long time arise, pull up a stool and shift your weight regularly – that is the only way that labor-intensive food like dumplings and meatballs are created by my hand in our kitchen.

Next issue to tackle: over-the-range microwaves that mandate lifting hot food above your head. Who thought this one up?

Babies

More daily tools that are too low? You betcha! It would appear babies are hard on backs all around.

I'll sing you the same song here as the dishwasher: Why is everything designed to be so low? We *know* better by now, humans. Babies are low when you put them on the ground because… well, because the ground is low and babies are small. So many baby-related props are unnecessarily low, though. The crib, the stroller, the changing table, the feeding table… My fused back hurts just *watching* my friends with their sore backs bending into their child's crib.

My back certainly voiced its protest after a few too many forward-bend, lower-down, lift-chunky-baby-out movements over a low crib. I wish I could bring that crib higher up. Work smarter, not harder.

How about always carrying a baby on *one* side, playing into your curves? Even if you're helping out a new mom and holding her baby on and off for an afternoon, it can awaken those imbalances if unchecked. Take it easy, take notes, and should the time come to set up your own baby furniture, you'll be ready to make it more back-friendly.

WISDOM AND STRENGTH

You are loved

Parents and caregivers are strong, loving beings who feel emotions very deeply – just like the rest of us. You as a patient are going through your own vortex of thoughts and feelings, but don't think for a second that your caregivers aren't going through their own vortex too. While you're trying to be easy on yourself, try to also go easy on them. They love you.

You may butt heads about things (what you want, what they think you should do). What you want is completely valid and be sure to voice how you're feeling, but don't dismiss their knowledge either – they probably have about 30 years' experience over you after all.

Your health *is* a big deal and is certainly serious enough to warrant all of the questions, tests, and appointments. Your family and friends want the best for you. They love you and want to help however possible. People are thinking of you and praying for you more than you can possibly know. If they're not sure how to help, ask for the support you need in the moment. If you're not sure what you need, a hug can be a great comfort. There's no maximum number of hugs to be given/received in a day!

In the event that you do not have a very strong support system at home, it certainly does not mean you don't deserve one or should go without one. Go online! There are tons of support groups and scoli warriors out there that would *love* to support you. (You'll find some in the "Resources" section at the back of the book.)

Empathy

While learning all about our bodies and health, we are simultaneously being treated to an education in empathy. Empathy isn't just concern or sympathy; it's understanding another person's feelings and experience without being told every single detail.[53] You may not know exactly what it's like in other people's shoes, but you feel similar emotions and pains. You now know precisely what it's like to have a day impacted by health. *You* wouldn't dismiss someone's feelings with a cool "You're fine"; you are sensitive to the challenges they face.

Since you know what actions help *you* out, you know what actions might be just what *others* need on a particularly rough day. You know what to say; you don't just jump in with a response, since you know the moment is really about emotional support and empathic listening.[54] You care and listen to the person, sincerely wanting to support them by being there – just like you appreciate being supported.

Professor Scoliosis makes us quickly appreciate that many ailments, like scoliosis, are invisible. You may not see a prosthetic limb under clothes. You may not know how much distress somebody's heart or stomach, diabetes or migraine is causing them. But you know what it feels like to struggle with something invisible and painful.

You also know you can't judge a person's inner being by how they look on the outside. This isn't just about scoliosis; this is a general life lesson about empathy in all situations.

Surprising people

"Some days are just tougher than others," thought every person ever at least once.

Nobody has a lifetime of *only* easy days with no worries or cares. *Everybody* has stuff. Our stuff just happens to be an extra, unique blend of ingredients layered atop the usual flavors of life. This special smoothie microdoses you into a mind frame of resilience and determination. Embrace it and thrive on it!

No matter which story you read within these pages – or experience in your own scoli-saga – you'll notice a theme of "never give up." To me, determination is being fed up but never *giving up*. May seem a tad military, but there's no benefit in "giving up." None.

People may automatically assume you're weak or frail due to your back "condition." They may suggest you take elevators instead of stairs, offer to carry your bags, or give you extra leg room on a plane. While that is all very considerate and caring – and yes, please, I love extra leg room! – you do not *require* all of that. Do you know why? Because your super smoothie of experiences has made you *so* strong.

You already know that, but other people may not know that yet. And therein lies yet another advantage: People will routinely be impressed by you! They have no idea what it's like to be in your body. They only know what it might be like through what they've heard in mainstream media (which, of course, offers a blatantly inaccurate caricature of scoliosis). To the average Joe, you should barely be able to walk or carry anything, let alone live life without a handicap parking permit.

Shock them. Awe them. Surprise them. All. The. Time.

In my late twenties, I finally made plans to ski the ultimate Canadian venue for an avid downhill skier: Whistler Blackcomb in British Columbia. This was the trip I had wanted to take my entire life, and I had saved up and planned it for months. I dreamt of carving those slopes with my friend, taking in the views, and being surrounded by fellow nature adrenaline enthusiasts. I was beyond ready and boarded the plane to Vancouver with the biggest grin plastered on my face.

Landing in Vancouver, I first stayed with family for a few days. Apparently the universe decided to take this opportunity to test my strength once again and, on day two, sent my lower back into a complete state of spasm. There was piercing pain in my back and legs, exquisitely unbearable day and night. The anger I felt was beyond words. Furious would be putting it mildly. *Of course* my back would throw ginormous wrenches into my ultimate dream experience and foil my ski trip plans! How *dare* it do this to me, especially since I had been *so good* with my self-care and exercises, and deserved some fun. I did *nothing* weird or stupid to bring this on. What was I supposed to do now? I was not at home near the security of my exercise props or physical therapists… How was I to make the road trip to Whistler, let alone *ski* the biggest hill of my life? These were all problems I had no answers for.

Part of me wanted to just *stop*. To give in to the break my back apparently wanted… which I likely would have done were I at home for this event. But giving up was not an option in the midst of a fun trip for "General Percy Veer" (my determined inner being), who forever refused to let her fused back stop her from living. I still had some time to sort this out before the drive to Whistler. So I took it one day at a time, using all the experience and knowledge I had accumulated to date to try to be kind to myself and fix this as best as possible before we hit the road.

By day four, I was only a smidge better. I was out for lunch with my family and had to take a short, steep flight of stairs down to the restaurant. I latched on to the handrail with white knuckles, taking one torturous step at a time, feeling sharp pain shooting through my lower back and into my legs with every movement. My whole left side seemed useless, but my fused spine was fine. I had known this sensation before. I felt ancient, broken, scared, and extra furious. But I took it slow, with some *very* deep breaths and cautious movement, flipping back and forth in my mind between, "You can do this, take another step!" and "Why is this happening to me?!"

What would having a breakdown in the middle of a restaurant gain me? Nothing. What would canceling my trip to Whistler accomplish? Nothing, other than lost non-refundable deposits and a "foiled" goal. I wanted some quality, serotonin-fueled fun! My family watched me sort this out, shocked that I was still going through with it. They were equal parts concerned and impressed.

And then my friend and I drove to Whistler. I took some emergency-reserve prescription painkillers to get me through that car ride. With that step completed, the universe issued *another* challenge to overcome: My rental skis were far too long and the boots were far too big. It was like navigating a canoe down a scary, unknown hill with steep surprise drop-off cliffs. Not that I needed any extra challenges, seeing as I was pretty much skiing with only the use of my right side, having little-to-no ability to leverage the muscles in my left hip and leg, and pain emanating all through my back.

Backs are strong, and so are we. Slow turns, early brakes, no moguls or jumps, strict conversations with my body to make it do what I required of it... and we did it (gracefully or not) without any ski-related injuries! We skied two full days, made full use of the hotel hot tub to massage those muscles, stretched before and after, and ended up having the time of our lives! I surprised my family and friends with this one, tackling it head-on when I could have easily bailed. I had learned enough about my body to know nothing was broken or needed emergency care – had that been the case, I would have ceased all plans.

We are enduring scoliosis every day, yet we are thriving and staying sane while *mostly* making it look easy. That is *incredible*. Keep it up! "Didn't think I could run that marathon because I have scoliosis? Let me color you surprised. Didn't think I could do the splits? Look at what I've been working on. Didn't think I could get a degree because the media has you believing I am Quasimodo? Check out this framed diploma. Didn't think I could hike the big mountains? One step at a time, baby. Didn't think I could ski the big mountains? *Swish, swish*. Had your doubts about my ability to land that big new account at work? Guess what, the client has back pain too and we talked about that for an hour."

We can do almost anything. Except maybe bungee jumping... but I don't want to do that anyway. Allow me to rephrase that: We can do almost anything we *want* to do, maybe a bit more carefully or differently because we're smart enough to know how to care for ourselves. And we'll do it while surmounting some steep physical odds. Go ahead and color people every shade of impressed!

Responsibility

Which would you rather be: Somebody who sits on the couch all week not bothering to do laundry, wash dishes, go outside for some fresh air, make dinner, or enjoy all the opportunities life has to offer? Or somebody who understands the value of time and exercise, is able to get chores done in no time, goes for a walk around the neighborhood to keep healthy, makes it on time to physio/massage/hospital appointments, *and* enjoys life to its fullest?

(Please tell me you picked the second option.)

If you are in high school and taking your scoli care seriously, you may become wise beyond your years in no time. I'm not talking about more wrinkles – I'm talking about figuring out what's important in life. Before I was diagnosed, I could easily lounge in bed until 11:00 a.m. on a Saturday, spend the afternoon watching TV, lob in a load of laundry to say that I crossed something off my list, and wait for Monday to show up. My diagnosis forced me to look at what my responsibilities were… while simultaneously piling on more. I had to learn to prioritize to keep my life balanced, since caring for my health was in my hands. I was responsible for doing my exercises at home, not my parents; I didn't need them holding my hand through it all each day.

Professor Scoliosis taught me the difference between a "must do," a "should do," and a "won't do today." The "must do" always includes movement of some sort: a walk in the morning, a stretch on the floor, scoli-specific exercises, maybe a visit to the gym. You are responsible for taking care of yourself.

You absolutely have to carve out time for your health *and* your regular human tasks when you've been given the part-time job of back maintenance. You *can* find a balance and achieve everything you want while feeling confident. Professor Scoliosis also gives many of us an appreciation for exercise – *not* to change the way you look but, rather, to take care of yourself. It's quite easy to stay motivated when the goal is to *feel* good instead of only to *look* good.

You're on your way to the real world, and you know what's truly important, including your health, your time, and your support network.

Deep appreciation for life

We all know that life moves fast. Blink a couple times, and the next thing you know, you're writing about scoliosis lessons. But life is wonderful! Have you ever paused to think about how staggeringly minuscule the odds of you being here, right now, experiencing this planet actually are? Tiny. Don't ask me for the actual math; this isn't that kind of book. Think about how many people are in your family tree. I know you don't know them all because they go back for generations. Think about how many people had to outrun bears, escape diseases, not starve to death, live long enough to have kids, meet your great-great-great-great-great-great-grandfather, survive childbirth to create your ancestors, and then keep them alive too.[55] Let's let that settle in your brain for a minute.

All of that and then some had to happen for you to be here today reading this. Due to all of those events, you get to experience life, love, family, blue skies, green forests, laughter, and the full range of human emotion. You get a chance to do something with your life, whatever that may be. You could sit at home staring at the walls, ordering in food, never choosing to let the sun warm your skin or experience the satisfaction of cooking something with your hands to present to the family table. Or you could travel to the ocean and go scuba-diving with colorful fish among coral reefs, appreciating how infinitesimally small their odds of watching you watch them are.

Take a look around you. This is the only spot in the universe (that we know of) where anything can live as bountifully. That is *never* something we should take lightly.

Many of us find it terribly sad when people with near-perfect health decide to throw that all away by using and abusing their bodies. Smoking, alcohol, constantly eating fast food, drinking sugar-laced soda, being inactive... Yet here we are, having done nothing to "deserve" scoliosis yet fully able to appreciate life and not take it for granted.

Tough moments in life make you appreciate the good. If you care enough to give it some thought, they can add a whole extra dimension to what life is. AIS may not be life-threatening, but it is life-altering, and it can certainly help you realize what is most important in your life.

The power to help others

You are part of a community now. You don't need to apply, and there are no membership fees. Should you choose to partake, there is a global community of scoliosis warriors ready to answer questions and be your cheerleaders. Other people with a "weird feeling in their pinky toe when it rains sometimes" do not get such a community... but you do! Look for scoliosis awareness groups, peer support opportunities, fundraisers, marathons, etc., that help boost research, promote public education, and support others with scoli.

You are now also aware of the basics of idiopathic scoliosis and know that nothing we do causes it, it can't be "cured," and the best thing we can do is stay active and catch it early. If your local schools have no scoliosis early detection screening programs in place, why not speak with the administration to see what it would take to set some up? Grade school isn't too early since children are hitting puberty earlier these days, but middle school isn't too late and high school is still a good catch. Maybe you'll help identify someone's scoliosis, catching it nice and early, and be able to make a difference in preventing the curves from progressing. Remember that many parents get blindsided by their child's diagnosis, especially if it doesn't already run in the family. Scoliosis education is important all around!

We are all constantly learning, and sharing those lessons can help others. Between the internet and an overall sense of community support, you have the opportunity to get involved in topics that matter to you while helping others whose shoes you were once standing in. Lots of bracers and fusioneers go on to support new warriors through many different channels. More and more organizations are setting up one-to-one peer support groups, question-and-answer sessions, and casual group meetings. These hangouts need leaders to guide the conversations and speak about personal experiences – that could be you! The young new warrior who is having trouble with her brace at school would probably *love* to speak to you and hear a familiar story. The warrior about to have surgery is just as scared as you were and would *love* to hear about all of the things you do every day with some titanium. Supporting others through a tough time is the ultimate way to give back to this community and encourage scoli conversation.

MIND AND MATTER

You know you have scoliosis

You know you have it. It's not something you can unlearn. And why would you even *want* to? But depending on what's going on in your scoli saga, your mind can decide to remind you of it at any moment. At times, it can seem like a great big shark is swirling around in your mind, ready to chomp out a pleasant portion of your day.

We may not talk about it all of the time or make it known to others that it's on our mind… but it is. The trick is to demote it to a lower-grade thought. It has done nothing to deserve the power to take over our days. This demotion can take time, so be patient. Eventually you will have trained that shark to be less and less powerful, turning it into a dolphin whose squeaks you'll only have to deal with on occasion.

You will notice that you feel better when you take care of yourself. Learning about your back, your nervous system, your mind, and how to exercise from a scoliosis therapist can be a big step in the journey of taking care of yourself. You *can* handle your own mind and body – don't let the scoliosis shark take charge.

And now... it's time to stop thinking about how tall we could have been if our spines hadn't curved.

You know you're not exactly symmetrical

Scoliosis has been described as a feeling of not being quite centered. It can make people look "visually uneven" and feel some awkward discomfort. (It's not always straight pain.) Other times, it can balance itself out on the inside and not show large imbalances on the outside when standing, but that discomfort can still be present. No matter what, scoliosis causes some asymmetry, and sometimes you can be super aware of it. (Hello, fellow perfectionists!)

Is one shoulder up higher than the other? Are you rotating forward to the left? Where is the concavity in the thoracic/lumbar? Does one arm swing more when you walk because your shoulder is out? Is a rib hump constantly grinding against waiting room chairs and park benches? Symmetry is lost in scoliosis. *You* know it the most, and of course *you* feel it the most.

Over time, you can learn corrective exercises that introduce more symmetry. These might be brand new topics for you that are made even more complicated since they are so very personal. Plus, you have to watch yourself in mirrors as you work to add symmetry to your body... which is not always something you want to be confronted with. That incentive to finally feel more centered is a hefty one, though!

Hard on yourself

It's incredibly easy to be hard on yourself when you have scoliosis. That's right, it's not just you! Scoliosis is at the center of your body and easily at the center of your universe. It can affect your body, your mind, and your social connections.

Have any of these thoughts crossed your mind before?

- *Arghhh!* I can't touch my toes today! I'm so broken.
- Can't believe the noise my brace made when I hit the side of that table. Everybody stared at me.
- I didn't do anything to deserve this *thing*. Why couldn't I just be *normal*?
- Oh great, it hurts to walk today. Guess I'll just sit down. *Arghhh*, it hurts to sit too? Really? Why, body, why?
- Ugh! My brain knows I could reach that pen on the ground. My fusion is just in the way.
- Look at that girl's outfit. It's so cute. I wish I could wear something like that! We have the same build… but I have scoliosis and it would probably sit funny on me.
- I don't want to go out with my friends tonight. My back is hurting and I don't want to be a burden.

So many scolis have echoed similar thoughts from their past; many very hard on themselves in the thick of it. Know what that means? That's right: *Many of us are hard on ourselves*. The saddest part here is that we don't need to be hard on ourselves *at all*. We're already going through enough. What does being a bully to yourself accomplish? Nothing good, that's for sure.

Scoliosis is a complex and multidimensional diagnosis; it should be treated beyond the physical side. Trauma doesn't just get over and done with. Psychologists can help break through the anger, shame, and sadness that can accompany scoliosis, whether during scoli treatment when young or later in adulthood.

The way you talk to yourself is very important. You *can* change a mindset from "Why do I have dumb scoliosis?" to "I'm going to do my scoliosis exercises today to help myself and improve, and that is *fantastic!* Excellent job! Good for you!" Then you can pat yourself on the back as a physical congratulations. That may sound corny, but it's actually a psychologist's tip!

Of course, simply being kind to yourself is much easier said than done. But it's worth it. It feels *so* much better than constantly mentally berating yourself.

Repressing trauma

Sadly, I don't remember chunks of my high school years while I was dealing with bracing and surgery decisions. I had to survey friends and dig out old pictures to fuel stories for this book. Good thing everybody these days takes 60,000 pictures a year, so that shouldn't be a problem for you guys anymore!

Scoliosis can bring stressful, tough, traumatic moments. Don't kid yourself if you can't remember them. Your brain tries to help out by making some of those memories less detailed and vivid. There are a ton of studies, opinions, and controversies out there about brains repressing or forgetting traumatic memories – a debate which I am not about to step into.[56] It may be a kind of self-preservation tactic so that you don't relive those moments in your mind over and over again. Perhaps your brain didn't like that then and doesn't want to see it again.

Most of this book is about how wild the body can be. But let me remind you that the brain is just as wild, if not wilder!

Beyond the physical

This darn scoliosis sure can play tricks on your mind. It's all too easy to get down in the dumps and feel hopeless or stressed. Sometimes your overall state of mind can get gray. Sometimes one little thing is the final straw to make you blue. Something as simple as sitting in a wooden chair and feeling half your ribs grinding painfully, crookedly against it. Or going to shave your armpits and noticing that one side is extra deep today thanks to a rotation and skewed shoulder blade.

Sadness pairs well with feeling alone. How many times did a simple headache launch you into a blue mood of hopelessness for the future? Even though you know you're going to have headaches all through your life. Even though you know, despite the pain, they're not life-threatening. Even though they're not a visible injury that everybody can see. Everyone at the school or office knows right away what it means when you say, "I have a headache." What's their immediate response? "*Oooh*, that sucks. I had one last week too. They can put such a dent in your day. Would you like some Advil? I know they can hurt pretty good sometimes."

There are a lot of parallels between a headache *ow* and a scoliosis *ow*: recurring, painful, not life-threatening, and invisible. And yet, if you told somebody, "My scoliosis is really hurting me today," they would not be able to relate as easily. Should you hazard an explanation, most still don't have any reference point to be able to understand the sensations you're enduring, leaving you on your own yet again.

Sadness pairs nicely with frustration too. How about the frustration that can build up while doing prescribed scoliosis exercises at home? Those exercises are not designed to be fun or fancy-free. Instead, they're often awkward and take an immense amount of mental energy to focus on. Not to mention they can sometimes hurt as you're working your body against itself, and that takes some practice. You can feel overwhelmed, fed-up, and discouraged, *especially* if you've been let down by practitioners before whose hard exercises didn't work. It can be a direct path to thoughts of "I hate this, I hate my body, I'm so exhausted, I'm done," which of course does nothing to help your pain.

What about the mental energy expended on scoliosis worries every day? Worrying about what to wear to cover some physical aspect you may not love yet. Worrying about what other people at school or at work might be saying. Worrying about finding a significant other who accepts your scoliosis. The effects of these thoughts can add up!

And then there are the questions about the future: "Will this ever get better? Will I ever feel 'normal'? Will I ever find a treatment and exercises that will actually help? Will bracing help? Will surgery help? Will anybody ever understand what I live with? What will happen as I age?" If not fused: "Are my curves going to worsen? How will my quality of life be affected? Will I ever need a walker?" If fused at a young age: "How will this affect pregnancy? What about labor and epidurals? What about complications?"

Stop. Breathe. That worrying route can make even the happiest clown see their world in greyscale. Part of this journey is about finding a way to come to terms with the situation. How can you possibly find peace with something you always wish was different? The first step to bouncing back is reminding yourself that you are *not* the only one dealing with this, feeling like this, or worrying about all of this. Feel a smidge better? Just because we are not speaking daily to other people who experience what we're experiencing, it doesn't mean they're not out there.

There are numerous mental and emotional side effects to scoliosis that are only *just* starting to be addressed. Those of us living with scoliosis know first-hand that they're linked. (*Everything* is linked!) Have you ever had a stressful day and noticed your shoulders tightening up? Psychology is finally beginning to be included in the "doctor + surgeon + physiotherapist" treatment equation of scoliosis, but it's only just beginning to make itself heard. Maybe someday, upon scoliosis diagnosis, a psychologist prescription will automatically come with the physiotherapist prescription (plus a box of tissues for good measure). Package deal, three-for-one special! Parents are not therapists, and carrying all of these pains and worries alone alongside you can be *exhausting* after a while. Speaking to a neutral, professionally trained person (even if you don't think you need anybody's help) can feel like a weight's been lifted off of you, *especially* if they know about scoliosis. There is *absolutely no shame* in talking to somebody, at any age. Give a chit-chat a try and see what comes up. We can *all* benefit from emotional support, even if we don't have scoliosis.

Crying

You're going to cry. Crying is a normal part of the human experience, especially for big life events such as this. It is totally okay and actually pretty cool that your body does this. Allow yourself to feel your feelings in a healthy way and let it all out; don't try and bottle it up.[57]

You may even notice different types of crying: slow tears; big sobs; salty, sad elephant tears; crying from frustration or being overwhelmed; crying from fear of the unknown; midnight tears on your pillow... I'm sure there's a scientist somewhere who has been studying these waterworks for years in a lab. You get firsthand experience!

Should the situation necessitate a tearful release of emotions after bad news or some sadness courtesy of scoliosis, let it happen! Tears also happen in support groups *all the time* when somebody opens up about a scoliosis challenge or worry – the whole room can be in tears in no time. And that's not a bad thing! Feel it. (It's probably a good idea to keep it together during the majority of your day-to-day life so as not to affect your school or work, though.)

When you can't touch your toes

Some days the ground can seem very far away. Even if you sit down to try to make it come closer, there's still quite a gap to get to the floor. Our household had both a fusioneer and an unfused scoli. There were days where *neither* of us were able to put socks on without a struggle or tears shed.

The piece of paper lying flat on the floor? The toy your kid wants picked up? The napkin that drifted off your patio table? Fused or not, you reach to grab it and then are starkly reminded that – *oops,* nope – that's as far as you go! Your brain may still think you can arch forward and reach the floor, especially from a seated position, but today's mad muscles will simply not allow it. Here's hoping you are naturally gifted in using your toes as fingers to grab small objects and kick them up to your hands.

All things considered, I tend to think that a person's feet are simply too far from their hands. It's clearly a design flaw! Feet and ankles are so very far away that you may begin to wonder how you ever got anything done with such incredibly long legs! When did popping on warm socks or boots become an Olympic event, complete with points for a hole-in-one and deductions for tripping over yourself? When did shaving ankles become a complex yoga session? Alas, your legs didn't lengthen overnight; your range of motion is merely being extra limited by some mad muscles.

Should you happen to be in such a toe-touch battle with your back at this moment, I feel for you. Truly and deeply. Be it pre-op, post-op, no-op, or braced... this can be infuriating! It is not a fun time, and your mind can become terribly sad, angry, and frustrated.

There is nothing to be gained from forcing yourself to the point of tears to pick up an errant pencil off the floor when your back is in spasm. Nothing at all. That pencil can stay down there for a little while. Hairy ankles are okay. People have no business inspecting your ankles up close anyway... or judging the volume of toys, napkins or writing implements lying around your house. Those who care about you are only going to care about helping.

One nuisance at a time – right now, the spasm gets priority. Leave the ground where it is and take some time to care for your health, whatever that may be. Maybe something calming, some myofascial release, massage, gentle walking, scoli exercises... how about a hot tub session?

Finally being able to touch your toes again

How much negotiating have you done with your back as you've struggled to touch your toes? The demanding: "Just let go!" The questioning: "Why won't you let go!" The begging (sometimes followed by the praying): "Please just let go." The giving in: "Well, guess this is how it is now." The fury: "STOP IT. JUST

RELAX." Frustration can build within until you start to wonder if you'll ever be able to manage a home pedicure again. It's all too easy to lose hope during this period, especially as the days add up. There's no kitchen timer counting down to let you know when you'll be freed from this seized state. It's not easy.

Nor it is easy to remind yourself that sometimes things just need time and care to heal. But then somewhere along the line, either out of the blue or from some form of treatment, you are able to move a little bit more. Breathe and sleep a little bit easier. Bend a little bit farther. No strain! No pain! Hello, little piggies! I've missed you.

This is a good thing! You can finally effortlessly shave your legs, put socks on in a second, and pick up the litter lying around on your floor. Days, weeks, or months of back pain have prevented you from being nimble and quick, instead waking you up at night, making you change plans and schedules. This release is wonderful news that can cause a flood of both elation *and* irritation.

Cue the waterworks. Here comes that overwhelming rush of emotions. Joy: "I can touch my feet and am released from my pain cage!" Frustration: "Why did I have to endure all of those hours of pain? Why?" A dash of pensiveness: "How can I all of a sudden touch my feet when I spent the last two months so far from them? Was this some lesson from the universe?" Mix it all up real good. It's almost like your brain doesn't know which thought or emotion to work through first, so it just bubbles over into an overwhelmed, elated state. How's that for a reminder that your unique back affects your life *and* that your emotions are valid?

Imagining what other people see

Walking into a crowded place, dozens of eyes around... who in here is going to see it? Can they tell? Do they see something different about me? Can they put their finger on it? What are they thinking when they see me walk/sit/bend near them? Has their opinion of me changed? Can they see my protrusions? Are they wondering why the middle of my back doesn't bend at all? Are my shoulder blades winging out a lot today? Is my mind just overthinking this? To the last one: yes.

Fused or not, these thoughts about other people may cruise through a scoli's mind now and again. Instead of checking in to see how you feel in that otherwise innocuous moment, you may think more about how *others* see you.

How utterly exhausting is that? How much energy could be saved by simply *not* entertaining the idea that you are some object to be objectified instead of the beautiful human you are? Think of all of the other important thoughts and fun conversations you could have instead. Take a moment to enjoy a nice dinner without thinking about the table next to you noticing your one bigger rib cage against your chair. Forget them! There is nothing to be ashamed of here! It's just another part of us that needs love and care, after all.

Nobody sees it as much as you do. Savor that fine meal, enjoy the moment, and conserve your energy for some honest-to-goodness fun. Everybody else out there is so consumed with their own lives and problems that even though you may think they're analyzing you, they most likely are not. Some of us go years with only our closest friends knowing about it, just because *we told them*.

What I gathered from all of my conversations for this book about self-perception and shame is that a funny thing seems to happen over time with many warrior elders: They stop caring what other people think. This may be something that comes with years of experience, but becoming at ease with your scoliosis instead of hiding it seems to be the healthiest route, if not always the most natural instinct.[58] Overall, other people's thoughts are not a worry to worry about.

Feeling normal most of the time

You wake up, stretch, eat breakfast, brush your teeth, go to school or work, hang out with friends and family, learn some life lessons, get promotions, cry over relationships, play sports, get upset about the state of the world, help your community, go on trips, bake a cake… It's completely possible to have a "normal" life with scoliosis. (Let's not get into the sociological definition of "normal" here.)

Since you can still do just about everything that a person with a straighter back can do, it's surprisingly easy to forget about it sometimes. And that's a great thing! It's not like you're cooped up for treatment day in and day out. (Although if you have a brace, I know it can feel like that at times.) Sure, you may have some days that are worse than others, but who doesn't?

Remember that *everybody* experiences pain. You are doing okay! Regardless of AIS, we can all complete post-secondary education, embrace careers in various fields, travel extensively, go on insane adventures with great friends, and meet the most incredible people along the way. Overall, *you* crush life more than AIS crushes you.

You can get used to anything

If you have to get used to something, you will. Wish all you want, but your old straight spine layout is not coming back, ever. You have no other choice here: Your body may have changed, but it is now your *new normal* to work with moving forward.

You will begin to recognize which shirts or dresses will definitely *not* sit well on your body just by looking at them on the hangers. You will get used to wearing a back brace all day and night. (Eventually you almost forget you're even wearing it.) You will figure out a desk and chair setup for your school or office that supports you in all the right places. You will get used to leaning a bit in one direction, noticing it, and actively correcting it with the guidance of a PSSE pro. You will figure out a way to fit a fusion through small car doors. You will devise plans to pick things up off the floor when you can't reach your feet. You will learn about what is happening with the muscles in your back. You will find exercises and treatments that assist you. You will figure out how to thrive with scoliosis.

You will get used to it all. Just give it time and never give up!

SCOLI INTERACTIONS

People not understanding what scoliosis feels like

Scoliosis doesn't always hurt, but it can certainly up the odds of having pain. One warrior with chronic pain used to think, "Do other people actually wake up *not* in pain? That can't be real." After her surgery alleviated all of her pain, she had a realization: "I didn't know what it felt like to *not* be in pain." For those of us in scoli pain, we can get a bit miffed when we read online that "scoliosis doesn't hurt." It most certainly can.

Pain can become a part of our world. When somebody else feels a similar back pain, it can put things into perspective. My high school friends were healthy, active teenagers who had never experienced great pain ordeals aside from a sprained ankle here or there. Many were athletic; a couple were fantastic dancers. The specifics at this point are hazy, but one of these friends somehow "threw out her back" mere days before the big school dance showcase and was unable to perform. She was lost as to what to do or how to endure it. "Heat? Ice? Acetaminophen? Ibuprofen? How can I sit, walk, move? How can something hurt so bad? Where is this coming from? Why did this happen? What can I do?" I vividly remember her standing at her locker, turning to look right into my eyes when we were alone, and saying, "I can't believe you feel like this every day. I am so sorry. This is awful, and I know it will go away for me. I don't know how you do it."

That was my first moment of realization that *nobody* knew what was going on in my body except me. Finally, somebody else in the school was experiencing similar pain to what I endured daily. These kinds of situations can give others a peek into the life of a person experiencing chronic back pain from ailments such as scoliosis. It certainly confirms that you're not "just complaining" about something insignificant. This could be the worst thing they've ever experienced, so sympathize with them. It's an opportunity to outwardly support while inwardly reminding yourself how strong you are every day.

You are the only person living life in your body. You certainly did not pick out this form for its superior design, but it's entirely yours to reside in. The same is true for every single being on this planet: Every body is unique. Imagine if we could switch bodies with people willy-nilly? That's some terrifying sci-fi situation in my mind's eye… let's not go there. Let's simply leave it at this: Nobody can ever completely know what another person's body is feeling at any given time. It is impossible.

Fellow scoliosis warriors will be able to commiserate with you the most. Seek out these people! Even though no two curves, backs, or pains are the same, the folks that have scoliosis know a thing or two about what you're going through. As for those with zero scoliosis experience or education, most seem to be more inquisitive than dismissive. They realize this is a medical condition and not something you can control. They may ask what the pain feels like, where it is, how a brace works, what the surgery was like… They want to know, even if they will never feel it themselves. These folks are also likely to say something caring, like, "I have no idea what you're going through, so you just let me know if I can help somehow." You may not yet be ready to provide those answers, and that's okay! Know that it takes courage to discuss it and time for outsiders to wrap their heads around it.

Then there are the completely clueless ones. These ones are extra tricky to communicate with about your situation, especially if they have no basic understanding of any chronic illnesses. These ones may say things, like, "Oh come on, there's no way it can be that bad." They may not mean any harm and are simply totally unaware of what you have going on. Keep an eye out for them and remember that they're not in your shoes. If you feel up to it, try to calmly provide some scoli information.

Physical and emotional feelings are complicated things to express, even to close family and friends. It can also be incredibly frustrating to have people doubt you or question your state of being. Difficult communication and difficult reception don't exactly go well together, do they? There's not much you can do about everybody else out there, so focus on what *is* in your control: Keep talking and keep your end of the communication going. Talk to your parents, siblings, friends, guidance counselor, psychologist... and keep trying to explain what's going on in your mind and body. It may seem like "extra work" but it's worth it – giving up and carrying it all on your shoulders alone gets so heavy after a while.

Remember how I dismissed the sci-fi narrative at the beginning of this section? Allow me to bring it back for a minute, because I would just *love* to pop those doubters into my form for a half hour and see how they would fare. No, I am *not* making a scene about tying my shoelaces for attention. Go ahead. You try to reach your toes today while in my body. I freakin' dare you. Yes, it *does* get annoying trying to correct your upper-right side forward and upper-left side backward, breathing into that upper left-side while *also* watching your lower-left and lower-right sections, pelvis, and head (or however your curves are set up). Have you achieved that alignment yet? Not so easy, is it? Now do that regularly. Forever. Ah, there, now you've found scoli compassion!

That would probably be the worst sci-fi movie ever, but it would certainly educate a bunch of people. Maybe it'll help you to know that almost everybody will experience back pain at some point in their life.[59] Still, our *ow* is legitimate. Be gentle with yourself when somebody questions it and keep talking about what it feels like. Seek out other people – those who know, know.

Unsolicited advice

Everyone has opinions and ideas. Many people have advice that they want to voice, thinking it might help you (whether or not you even asked for said advice).

A common tidbit of advice non-scolis offer scolis is "Oh, you have a bad back? You should definitely talk to a doctor!" Yes, thanks, I haven't done that ever… Or how about "Have you ever tried *this* magic treatment?" Once again, yes, thank you. Almost guaranteed that I already considered it.

These situations become easier when you remind yourself that *people generally mean well*. They're not offering up their advice to try and make you feel worse; they're offering advice because they genuinely think there may be a chance you could use it to your advantage. But yes, it can get annoying being on the receiving end of that constantly, especially when it's for something sensitive or traumatic.

Take it or leave it, try something new if your interest is piqued, and laugh off the rest. In all my years of receiving unsolicited back advice, not once was any PSSE guidance supplied – now *that* would have been welcome advice. Big exhale of annoyance out, deep breath of common sense in.

Telling your new significant other

When you're in the fresh honeymoon phase of a new relationship, it's sunshine and rainbows and bliss. *Ahhhh*, the best feeling possible! As you get to know each other, the conversations start being about more "serious" topics like politics, religion, future plans, kids, and health. It turns out being self-conscious about scoliosis when getting close with somebody new – both for the "health" conversation and for closeness – is a common worry among the scoliosis community. Some decline massages if "the scoliosis conversation" hasn't been had to explain what "it" is yet.

The health conversation can be emotional and difficult at the start, but it gets easier. There's no right or wrong time to share your back story – it's entirely up to you. The very first step is building confidence with yourself and finding peace with your scoliosis. That in itself can take a while, depending on your back saga. Once you bridge that relationship with yourself, building trust with your partner will make the explanation even easier. The right person will care immensely about your health and wellbeing; anything less than support should not be acceptable – it's a relationship red flag!

Scoliosis can affect a relationship if it's already affecting *you* emotionally, mentally, and physically. As you merge your home with somebody else, all aspects of your lives become merged. However, your significant other should not be too affected – scoliosis is not contagious and partners should support each other through all aspects of life anyway. If you're gearing up for your first scoli conversation, set some boundaries for yourself in advance. Know where *your* comfort level is. Your significant other doesn't need to know every single detail right away if you don't want to offer up that information. They certainly won't understand it all right away, unless by some fluke they already know somebody with scoliosis. Even then, the odds of that person having the same back resumé as you are slim to none.

Remember: Everybody has "stuff." Allergies, anxiety, glasses, troubled pasts, heart conditions, stomach conditions, foot conditions, eating conditions, lack of empathy, a crippling fear of clowns... all kinds of stuff! No body is "perfect"; we are all human.

A scoli in the wild!

I see you, fellow scoli! I'd know that slanted neckline anywhere. I see myself in your shoulder blade. It's like looking in a mirror, and it's *great*!

Should we chat about it, becoming best friends? We could laugh at scoliosis-only things like small car doors, scars, and the heat of a back brace in the summer. Should I approach you and say, "Scoliosis?" to which you *might* reply, "Scoliosis!" We must have so many inside jokes all ready to go.

Probably best not to engage. But I see you, maybe you see me, and we're reminded that we're not on our own in the world with scoliosis. There are scoli warriors *hidden in pain sight* all around, and we don't even need words to identify with each other's strength.

EXTERNAL FACTORS

The "idiopathic" in "idiopathic scoliosis"

If you've taken a gander online at some scoliosis chit-chat, you may notice that many people are casually describing their own scoliosis with things like "I think it's genetic? I don't know. The spine curves. It just kinda happens."

This isn't an ailment that we have a clear and informative description for, for a couple of good reasons. First, there is no definitive known cause. Unlike developing lung cancer from clearly being a lifelong cigarette smoker, AIS is more involved. Yes, we do know that there is likely a genetic component that plays into its development.[60] However, many people who have zero known scoliosis cases in their family trees and are otherwise perfectly healthy still appear with curvatures. Why? Well… we're not totally sure. Researchers are working on that equation, but it takes time, money, and pressure.

Which leads to the second reason: It is complex. It's going to take a lot of research in many fields to decipher those complications and understand why it happens.

I've had moments of statistical curiosity about my own AIS, wondering where it fell within the numbers. Turns out finding easy-to-understand statistics that non-doctors can actually decipher on AIS per country, gender, age, race, and curve degree from a reliable source isn't easy. Nor are stats or visuals for degree of curvature versus pain, or the average height/weight at AIS diagnosis. In comparison, just about every piece of data imaginable is instantly and readily available for lung cancer statistics.

There are quite a few medical journal articles online about *this* curvature progression study or *that* symptom comparison, or even bracing and its relation to self-esteem. It's *wonderful* to see these studies happening for scoliosis, gaining any ground possible to find out what's going on. But their minute details can get *way* too scientific for the average scoli reading it at home, and the reader has to ensure the study is truly comparing apples to apples. It would be even *more wonderful* to start reading concrete explanations with crisp, colorful graphs and explanations in non-medical speak, not just "there might be a link between symptom A and curvature B." We are all eagerly awaiting the journal that says,

"AIS is absolutely caused by X, Y, and Z"! I cannot wait to see the "idiopathic" removed from AIS.

It's no wonder scolis don't always have an elevator pitch ready when given an opportunity to educate the surrounding population and further the quest for early detection. Many parents whose children are freshly diagnosed with scoliosis are initially at a complete loss or think that it's some kind of cancer.

Here's what we do know: Scoliosis is three-dimensional and not just a side-to-side bend. You do not create idiopathic scoliosis within yourself by wearing heavy backpacks, but adding lopsided weight to an existing scoliosis case will not help it. There is no known total prevention, no magic vaccine – the closest thing to it is early detection. It cannot be cured; there is no medicine to straighten out the spine on its own. Research is underway to find out different avenues of causation. And finally, we know it can be *very* frustrating living with a medical diagnosis whose cause is still unknown.

The genetic component

An ailment that sometimes appears to be genetically transferred but whose causes are complicated and still not fully understood. Not much peace of mind for us when it comes to thinking about our future offspring, is it?

Sometimes it appears to be carried through the family tree. But even if there is no history of scoliosis in the family, it can still develop.

We could noodle on this and fret and worry about the what-ifs of our own future generations for days on end… but what would be the point? You *cannot* control the future. You *cannot* decide to have a child with no medical ailments. You *cannot* stop your life because of fear.

What you *can* do is continue to learn about scoliosis. You *do* know what it's like to experience scoliosis and what to screen for in your children early on. Just take it one generation at a time.

Modern medicine

Take a pause and think about how much has gone into scoliosis research, braces, and surgeries over the entirety of human existence. Answer: a lot. For a quick flip of perspective, consider a world with no understanding of how curves progress, or how rough this surgery could have been in the early days.

We first have to go back to the Greeks, as early as the Classical era in the fifth century BC. These guys were clued in to the science of scoliosis – theorizing, experimenting, and designing contraptions to try and correct spinal curves. The word "scoliosis" was even coined by the Greeks. Skipping ahead to the Early Middle Ages (aka the Dark Ages), there were other priorities at play, which saw a slowdown in scientific developments and progress. The main scoliosis belief seemed to be that "deformities" were essentially mystical payback for being "bad."[61]

Eventually, things started to pick up again. The first attempts at surgical spinal correction were in 1839 by a French surgeon named Jules Guerin. More than 1,300 patients received fusion with apparently mixed results, ending in a great big lawsuit. Nobody bothered with spine surgery again until the 20th century, around the time X-rays became available. Being able to peek at the spinal structure and curves allowed surgeons to think up new ideas. This era saw many more medical advances in this field and trials of new types of surgical procedures with varying results. Patients were typically immobilized for months after the operation. Some didn't hold the spinal correction, some didn't fuse, and others developed infections.[62]

In the early 1900s, after years of cumulative discoveries and advances, they came up with the idea to use bone grafts from the patient's tibia to help fuse the spine. It turned out that this didn't hold the surgical correction for too long, but good try… cue more scoliosis ideas into the mid-20th century! The "Cobb angle" became the standard in measuring coronal curves. The "Milwaukee brace" was designed and used for decades. In 1955, the "Harrington rod" was devised for spinal fusions. With a few more added contributions from the medical community, Harrington rods were the go-to until the late 1980s.[63]

Also consider the state of the hospitals, machines available, infection rates, brace fittings, test runs of new techniques that may or may not work, and recovery time for big-time surgery back then. No thanks! Incisions were not precision cut with technologically advanced tools either, and scars could look quite gnarly. Double no thanks!

It may have taken a *longggg* time to get where we are today, but we live in the era of science and technology. There is *so* much going on in the world of orthopaedics. Centuries of medical advances and stop-and-go research have brought us to the present, with new brace designs, new materials, new surgical techniques, new studies, more data... We may have a lot more to learn, but we don't have to walk through all of those discoveries once again at square one.

It's hard to imagine a world without all of the technological advances we get to benefit from in this lifetime. Not having the luxury of seeing bones via X-ray machine is unthinkable! How about low-radiation X-ray machines, computerized axial tomography (CAT), and magnetic resonance imaging (MRI), which are now all available? Beams of light can measure alignment, posture, tilt, and center of balance to help in treatment planning. Here we are, and we're never going back! Ask your parents about some of the orthopaedic methods available a couple of decades back, when they were exactly your age. You might just be flabbergasted at the technology they tell you about. But it took all of those stepping stones of invention to get us to where we are today.

Don't give all of the limelight to the "big" machines and tools, though. There is also research going into the *why* of scoliosis. Why more women than men? Why some girls during a growth spurt and not others? Why are some painful or pain-free? Does it have anything to do with certain hormones, vitamins, or minerals like manganese?[64] What about genetics? There are studies on a few genes that may play a role, most notably CDH7.[65] These questions need answering too! Imagine if we could get solid answers for these questions. We could increase early detection and prevention, and decrease pain, treatment, and surgery. That's the dream...

Have faith in other people, even if it is frustrating that we don't have all of the answers *now*. Some folks really are working to make this experience as pain-free and noninvasive as possible. It may not be moving at lightning speed, but it *is* moving ahead. Some people devote their entire lives to studying scoliosis, making advances, creating new braces, devising new surgeries, understanding pain, working on new exercises and treatments. Heck, some of my dearest healthcare practitioners and instructors went into their respective fields *because* they or somebody close to them had scoliosis. Not everybody can change the world, but each contributor is certainly making an impact towards helping others like us.

Internet research

Careful here. The internet can go from good to bad in a millisecond. When I was initially looking online into what this scoliosis thing was years ago, I was treated to horror stories and nothing but bad news. And then the pictures on the page would load… treating me to an extra visual of graphic surgical pictures that I *most certainly did not ask for.*

Today the internet is an even bigger space: a limitless universe of content that can pull you in for hours and hours with contradictory information and no end or hope in sight. Tread lightly. The natural tendency is for people to gravitate towards the worst information, like rubbernecking at a car crash scene. "What's going on? What's the worst that could happen? I need to know everything so I'm most informed and can worry about it all!"

No, you don't.

The internet absolutely has valid, informed, supportive information. (There's some listed under "Resources" at the end of the book to start you off.) Then again, the internet may prove completely useless in getting you correct information for your situation. If you search "Why does my shoulder blade stick out?" you are treated to an entire set of results about different disorders and nerve issues… not a single mention of scoliosis.

The online world can be unnecessarily scary or unvetted, containing incorrect information. You likely don't have the world's worst case of scoliosis, so don't psych yourself up for that with the help of the ever-willing internet.

Dig a little into scoliosis details, should you feel so inclined, but don't push yourself to the point of fear and tears. I got in too deep a couple of times with outdated surgical procedures and spent many nights wide awake with worry – which was completely unnecessary. Leave the professional care to the professionals, while remaining an advocate of your health. Get to the point of being knowledgeable enough to be able to ask informed questions of your healthcare professionals – and to make sure they *are* qualified professionals. Discovering other treatment options, hospitals, or brace technology available out there is the good stuff. It's cool having so much information at your fingertips online, but be sure to also *talk* to other people who have firsthand experience.

Then again, maybe you're a medicine enthusiast and want to dig through scientific reports with step-by-step details of surgeries. Hey, if that's your joy, go for it! We had one family member who was such an enthusiast and could not devour enough data. It was nice knowing somebody was well read on the topic, but the rest of us certainly couldn't stomach it.

An additional caution about social media while we're online. It can absolutely bring scoli warriors together as a community and provide a space to share stories, tips, and support. But it can be a blessing and a curse: tons of supportive images, with tons of potentially incorrect medical advice. Focus on the social media accounts that can help you at this moment.

Media

Where would we be without the good ol' media telling us how to look and feel.

Health is just *not* something to poke fun at. People live with all kinds of ailments with varying degrees of severity. And while scoliosis is not the worst of the worst, a bad case of it is definitely not the easiest of the easiest. It is life-altering *before* you even get to its social ramifications. In this modern day of a growing awareness and effort towards more inclusive and respectful content, how has scoliosis seemingly escaped the new standards?

Some of us were caught off guard by a graphic scoliosis depiction in a fantasy TV show. A female character was shy and unwashed, hair unkempt, no makeup, hunched forward and to the side (clearly having spinal curves and rotations). How did she choose to make herself more acceptable in society? Certainly not by washing up and developing some social skills, oh no. Off to a wizard for a lengthy, brutal, vivid, excruciatingly painful session of witchcraft and surgery to straighten out her spine (during which she insisted on being kept awake). Shiny tools and gore, red and white muscle and bone CGI'd across the screen, a woman's face contorted in pain. It completely caught the fusioneer viewer with trauma unprepared.

Her next appearance showed her standing perfectly upright with full makeup and a fancy hairdo, mesmerizing a room full of people with her radiance. Wait... what? The writers completely skipped past making this character go through any other adjustments whatsoever as a first step!

How about we don't falsely teach young women that their spinal curvatures are *all* that people see when they look at them? Or that a *straighter spine* is going to fix all of her problems? How about, in a society that is supposed to be more and more accepting, we actually *act* on that inclusion and write stories with our audience's well-being in mind? How about we don't trigger panic attacks in fusioneer viewers? How about we do *all* of that?

Let's set the bar here: I have not watched every single TV show episode and movie in existence. I am also not going to set out to accomplish that even to support education for this book. That's also far too much sitting (and I'm clearly not a fan of that). However, I have watched a diverse set of content and enlisted friends and the scoli community to report back on any scoliosis instances they come across. (Thank you all!)

Sitcoms tend to make light of the medical nature of scoliosis with mentions of chiropractors, imbalances, and the mumblings of "scoliosis" here and there for some cheap chuckle. All of those are lighthearted prime-time shows that are supposedly fun for the whole family. Mentioning scoliosis is a *good* thing – normalizing this condition and talking about it is important! But then some of these shows casually mention cases of childhood scoliosis and back braces to mock a character or detract from their qualities. It's a sort of visual shorthand to depict someone as being needy, uncool, or socially awkward. That's *not* so good.

And then there are darker humor shows that devote complete episodes to the theme of scoliosis, but with *zero* education included. They're all about making scoliosis and back braces hideous and making it socially acceptable to ridicule them. Those shows may argue that "nobody is safe" as they make fun of anything and everything, which is the type of humor they're going for and target audience they're appealing to.

There are a couple of movies out there that actually take scoliosis seriously. Alas, the scoliosis theme does not continue throughout the entirety of those films or involve itself in the ultimate outcome of the protagonist's journey. Romance and other drama comes into play, with scoliosis only a brief blip in the plot. A dash of normalization here, a scathing joke there, a nice attempt at a scoliosis story run over by another storyline...

Some good movements are happening, but they are few and far between. Back in 2002, a British theater company swapped the title *The Hunchback of Notre Dame* for *The Bellringer of Notre Dame*. Times have certainly changed since that story was originally written in 1831.[66] More recently in 2021, a kids' TV show included a character who told a friend she had worn a back brace for scoliosis in the third grade. This exchange strengthened the burgeoning friendship. Now *that's* what we want to see! You may also notice a fusion scar in a scene or advertisement where fusioneer actresses and models are baring their backs to the camera. That feels like seeing an extended family member on TV!

Social media can sometimes fill the need for more scoli representation, but it also comes with millions of scoli-free bodies, mean jokes, and incorrect medical advice that can have a detrimental effect. The strong visuals that have been created and distributed through all forms of media (including social media) over the years contribute a huge part of the public's perception of scoliosis today. More often than not, that visual is a caricature of a human bent every which way, inevitably mocked for being different, and not living life to the fullest. In fact, scoliosis is as real an illness as any other and deserves the same degree of sympathy, respect, care, and research.

Maybe somebody will depict a story on-screen about the true trials of scoliosis in today's world. Of wearing a back brace 20-plus hours a day in every type of weather. Of the small but numerous changes to daily life a surgery brings. Of the woes *every* scoliosis warrior endures and of the strength, resilience, determination, and compassion they develop. Something to showcase that we are *so* much more than our Cobb degrees. To depict the champion athletes, musicians, doctors, models, students, thinkers, entrepreneurs, moms, and dads with scoliosis that excel in whatever they set their minds to.

I want to see that movie. I want to see what you all conquer every single day, and I want the next generation of warriors to know, right at their diagnosis, that they too can conquer any challenge that comes their way. Imagine a visual story that a young scoli can *see* to prove this is not the end of their world but, rather, the start of a new education. Something for which you can press "play" on a low day and be reminded of your inner strength when you just don't have the energy to remind yourself anymore.

We are all incredibly strong, despite how TV, movies, and social media may depict us. We know it, our friends and family know it, and with continued hard work, more and more people will come to understand it. *Never* give up. *Always* take care of yourself. You are not alone.

DEAR PARENTS, READ THIS

Scoliosis has never been a "fun" diagnosis for a parent to hear. It's a serious medical condition with largely unknown origins that develops in children. Are you a parent or caregiver yourself, reading this to get some kind of insight as to what to expect? It's entirely normal for you to worry or feel lost. As I've said to all the scolis reading this book: *You are not alone*. If you go online, you may notice most online scoliosis community posts and questions are written by parents seeking advice, answers, or reassurances.

Dear Parents: We hear you too. You are in this just as deep, if not deeper, than your child. It can be overwhelming for everybody involved!

First of all, take a deep breath. *Nothing you did caused this*. AIS is not from sleeping funny, allowing bad posture, or buying the wrong backpack.[67] If your child is still quite young and you are simply getting prepared for a potential future scoli diagnosis, keep an eye on them for scoli symptoms early on (uneven shoulders, hips, ribs, pain in the shoulders or back), but don't stop checking until they're totally done growing. Many curvatures are discovered during summer months while swimsuits are in use, but keep checking the rest of the year. Be sure to mention any scoliosis family history to your pediatrician to ensure early and consistent screening.

If you are new to the scoli diagnosis, welcome. Try to steer away from feelings of guilt if your side of the family tree happens to contain another person with scoliosis. While you're at it, dismiss any guilt about not identifying it sooner – both are very common yet of no help to the situation at hand. You now officially know better than to simply dismiss all back pain as "growing pains," and as long as you're being supportive, you are doing great!

Young people diagnosed between 10 and 14 years old are not yet emotionally mature enough to fully comprehend what their diagnosis means, let alone find therapists. It falls to their caregivers to do the bulk of the research about next steps and options. You're in this together! There is going to be some trial and error in figuring things out; there is no set manual as every case is different. Information is the strongest thing on your side. Read as much as you can about scoliosis structures, treatment options, the overall nervous system, how to create genuine connections with your child, and how to create safe spaces. Look for pain management tools and methods, and scoliosis-specific therapy that includes education about your child's own body, psychological support, and fitness options. Remember that there are more options than only braces or surgery *and* that scoliosis can affect much more than just physical health.

There are *many* gaps between healthcare providers and patients, by the way. The simplest example is how focused the medical space is on the *physical* side of scoliosis without providing immediate support for the resulting *emotional* needs. The scientific community still needs to step up to address the connection between the physical bends and emotional impact, and create multidisciplinary teams that address this gap. (But that's not your personal mission right now.)

What else can you do to help? Talk. Talk. Talk. At a minimum, remember that you *do not know* what's going on in your scoli child's mind, and they *do not know* what's going on in yours. The only way to understand each other is to chit-chat regularly and connect. Maybe not all the time and through every dinner – keep some scoli-free normalcy – but make time for it. Car rides are a nice, casual setting. Going for evening walks or doing home workouts together can bring you closer and provide rich conversation time. You love them, they love you, but that's not enough to prevent missed communication and crossed signals. Avoiding a "broken telephone" situation takes a smidge more work – and, oh boy, is it ever work. Do your best to encourage communication and create a feeling of safety, where your warrior can *know* that it's safe to share what's happening in their world. The other half of this is *listening*. Don't try to solve the problem, make it all better, downplay their feelings, or deny what they're saying. Be in the moment and preserve that trust and safety.

Maintain that emotional support through every facet of this journey. Talk with your child who has been diagnosed, but don't forget to speak with their siblings. Should this proceed to bracing or surgery, the whole family should be involved as one supportive unit. Giving your support is *the number one thing* you can do. You can provide them with all of the material support possible, but the importance of also providing emotional support cannot be understated.

Every fusioneer I spoke to whose parents or caregivers stayed with them through the entire hospital stay expressed how they could not have done it without their physical and emotional support. This saga certainly has its ups and downs, and the never-ending support of family is the best medication available. Imagine waking up in a hospital room in the middle of the night, in pain, in an unfamiliar environment, unable to easily get out of bed on your own, knowing you just underwent something big. Wouldn't you want to be able to look over and see one of your parents in the lounge chair next to you? Can you imagine being completely alone? Just. Be. There. Get a dog-sitter, house-sitter, baby-sitter, whatever you need for your other responsibilities… but be there to support your child through appointments, crises, surgeries, and general scoliosis discussion.

And then talk some more. Talk about scoliosis with other parents and educators. I can't even begin to count how many conversations I've been a part of where the entire dialogue is at a normal tone and volume, but there is a hesitation every time before the word "scoliosis" is *whispered*. Seriously? Why is this "the ailment that shall not be voiced at regular volume"? You may not think you can do much to counter a social stigma, but it has to begin somewhere and the scoli community is a great group to get that normalizing ball rolling! One less person who leans in to this stigma is one more person who knows that this is not a "curse" that should be whispered but, rather, a serious, sometimes painful ailment that needs to be much better understood.

We're still not done talking. Another way to show support, get answers, fill in gaps from medical appointments, and facilitate conversations is to find other people who have undergone the same diagnosis, bracing, or surgery. Your child may not necessarily be bold enough to go out and find such a contact, so take the initiative to find a friend of a friend, daughter of a coworker, or local scoliosis support group that your child can speak with honestly. If your child is shy, one-on-one may be the way to go. If they're outgoing, then try out a support group. These are great ways to begin normalizing conversations about scoliosis outside of home or a doctor's office, answer worries or questions, be reminded that none of us are alone, and show that other people have lived successful lives with scoliosis!

Don't be shy about speaking with other scoli parents too – they have tons of information to share from their own experiences. It's also important for scoli parents to lean on each other for support.[68]

Maybe your child isn't very chatty. That's okay! Encourage them to keep notes or a journal on how they feel. Maybe not daily because that can be a lot on top of regular schoolwork and exercises – it shouldn't be a chore. But whenever they feel particularly happy or sad, or if something scoliosis-related happens, encourage them to "get it out" and jot it down. You, as a parent, can keep notes too. You are likely experiencing many feelings and fears, all of which are valid. You have much more on your plate, and it's also good for you to get it out of your mind and onto paper. The teenager is tough on any parent, let alone when something like scoliosis is challenging you further. Maybe someday you'll both be ready to read your journals as a way of putting those roughest scoliosis days behind you... or maybe not.

Whatever you do, *do not* nit-pick your child's body courtesy of scoliosis. Don't worry about the aesthetics of a shoulder being higher or one rib poking out more than another. Do not make them self-conscious about it. They're beautiful the way they are! Focus instead on calming your own stress; lowering their self-esteem will do nothing to help this situation. Nor will over-managing bracing or constantly correcting posture – it can work against that genuine connection and safety that is so important. Teenagers also need to create their own identities and become adults. Encourage extracurriculars and activity with friends instead.

The good news? You will come out of this a very close family. Aside from acknowledging the importance of family support, scoli patients often point out how this made their family very tight-knit. Even divorced parents have made peace and worked together to care for their child through scoliosis. It will not be sunshine and rainbows while you're in the thick of it, but hang in there. There is no parenting handbook that will tell you exactly what to do in every unique situation you encounter (in regular life and in scoli life). Just do your best, talk, and *be there*. If you're reading this, you're already doing great: You're searching for information! Keep going and remain supportive.

And finally, a note from my own mother: "You have to be positive, no matter what. Look for information. Trust that the hospital teams are always doing their best and what will happen, will happen. You could walk across the street today and be run over. No point worrying about everything in the future. Just stay positive and support any way you can."

THE BENEFITS OF POSITIVITY

There's no question about it: Life is not a walk in the park. It can be an obstacle course of spikes and mud, with ninjas throwing things at you and something definitely on fire somewhere. If you're running full throttle through that course without thinking and stopping to recharge, you're bound to fall into a deep pit without so much as a plastic spoon to help you get yourself out. Things can get pretty grim in that pit if you don't watch it. You can hear people above you running by and befriending the ninjas, maybe spraying down a couple of fires with a hose. But that's not you – you're not stopping and recharging – you're furiously digging yourself out of the pit and your first tactic is to throw a fire extinguisher *at* a fire (which *spoiler alert* does not put out the fire but makes it explode violently).

It is all too easy for life to get you down if you let it, and you get the added bonus of having a non-standard body. Here's where you get your education on positivity: You don't want to fall into that dark pit. You may look at it from time to time, but you are going to develop all kinds of techniques that work for *you* to get up, over, and around it.

It may sound corny (since it's constantly stated in self-help and self-improvement messages), but if you think you can or think you can't, *you're right*.[69] A negative state of mind can make the world seem bleak, but a positive state of mind can work wonders. It really is that simple. But, of course, it's *so* much easier said than done. How do you even start doing that, especially if you're a self-proclaimed "pessimist" or "realist"?

Here's a simple one to noodle on: I used to think of my back brace as a "stupid, hot, useless *insert preferred curse word here* hunk of plastic." I called it a "necessary evil" as I stared it down before putting it on for the night. What did that accomplish, really? Nothing other than infuriate me more and build upon that deep-seated hatred. I thought it was the worst thing to ever happen to me, so I was right. I had annoying metal braces for my teeth at the same time, but I didn't scowl at those daily even though they took a ton of cleaning and could cause pain. I never spoke to my orthodontics using such colorful terms while they were also working hard for me and were in the best interest of my health.

Something in my mindset had to change... and it eventually did. But it wasn't an overnight change or an "ah-ha" moment. It was gradual, and it took a lot of training for me to make myself pause when I noticed a negative thought. I learned to consider those thoughts, see what they were contributing to my situation, and assess whether my situation really was that dreadful. Given that pause and reflection, 99 percent of the time it turned out to be not so bad after all. Those are the opportunities to consider things in a different light.

My back brace (to continue that example) was no longer termed a "necessary evil" but, rather, a "necessary nuisance." The brace was temporary, after all, and it was doing its best to try to help me, as were all of the people involved in making it and treating my back. All I had to do was wear it or, as I called it, "brace bravely."

A positive mindset can truly improve your outlook on life. Never give up on helping your health and furthering your education. Keep yourself open to communication, and be honest about how you're feeling. Bad, low, or painful days are still likely to happen, but knowing it's temporary and knowing how to take the best care of yourself is empowering.

And here you are, working towards all of that. Chin up, fresh air, friends, family, exercise, comfy clothes, warrior community... take a great big, deep breath that you are here and can untangle yourself from any curve life throws your way!

Conclusion

I don't know you. I don't know what your diagnosis is, what your treatment plan entails, or what your social demands are. But I *do know* that you chose to read this to help yourself or a loved one through a very confusing and scary time.

So maybe I *do know* that you are inquisitive and caring. That's wonderful! I sincerely hope you continue to take the time to care for yourself and others, and learn throughout.

I wrote this as the book I wish I had access to when I was freshly diagnosed, dealing with a brace, feeling completely different, lost beyond words, and facing surgery. I had no other stories or experiences to look to for tips or support. There is so much I know now – having learned it all the hard way – that I wish I knew then.

This book is my contribution to make sure *all* warriors know the following is true: You are not the only one dealing with 3-D spinal curves and the resulting emotional ups and downs. You can absolutely handle this, with some extra information and support.

Take care of yourself and your back.

Acknowledgements

My heartfelt appreciation to the following people for their time and willingness to discuss their experiences with me. Your honesty and openness was heartwarming, as is your support of this book:

Dr. Peggy Baxter, Katelyn Carlson, Lily Clark, Kyra Condie, Abby Cunningham, Elisabetta D'Agata, Simone Dimas at Pillow Pod, Megan Glahn Castille at Scolios-us, Emily Hale at Build & Breathe Scoliosis, Lauren Higginson at Higgy Bears, Abby Kraai, Alia Leonard, Claudia Lepp, Carmen Lynch, Stacey Mears at Brace Buddies, Dr. Jean Ouellet and the Canadian Paediatric Spine Society, Kat Sherrie, and Katherine Southard.

Thanks to my professional editor who helped transform my wild manuscript about wild spines into this final product.

My compliments to the online scoliosis warrior community who support each other daily, through good times and bad. You are an immense source of inspiration.

Absolute gratitude to my parents and my best friend for helping me stand up tall through years of scoliosis. Special mention to Betsy for cruising with me through it all.

Resources

Books

- *A Consultation with the Back Doctor* by Hamilton Hall, MD
  The third book from one of the world's foremost back surgeons. While not scoliosis-specific, it explains the back's structure and resulting pains in a question-and-answer format.

- *Braced* by Alyson Gerber
  A contemporary novel about scoliosis, this middle-grade reader offers insight into what it feels like to have scoliosis and a brace.

- *Deenie* by Judy Blume
  A novel from 1973 about a young girl's struggles with a scoliosis diagnosis, a Milwaukee brace, family, and friendships.

- *Enjoy Life with Idiopathic Scoliosis During Adolescence: Psychology for Professionals of Scoliosis* by Elisabetta D'Agata
  A practical tool for healthcare professionals and educational resource for scolis and their families. Provides strategies and creative ideas to help scolis find the path of resilience.

- *Growing Up in a Brace: Notes of My Scoliosis* by Kaisa Virolainen and Marja Heinonen
  The perspectives of both mother and daughter through almost twenty years of scoliosis appointments, treatments, and emotions.

- *Scoliosis and the Human Spine* by Martha C. Hawes, PhD
  A thoroughly researched review of modern approaches to scoliosis treatment, this book clearly explains common terms to readers while proposing changes to the management of scoliosis.

- *The Silver Horned Girl* by Lisa Owens
  A children's book to help with anxiety and self-confidence of dealing with scoliosis and bracing. Its messages can be appreciated by people of all ages.

- *Why Do I Hurt? A Patient Book about the Neuroscience of Pain* by Adriaan Louw
  Explains the science of pain in plain language – what it is, how it works, and the connection to the central nervous system.

Online learning

- *Ahead of the Curve* **Podcast:** thescoliotherapist.com/podcast
  A podcast hosted by certified Pilates instructor and Schroth method physical therapist Dr. Meghan Teed.

- *Behind the Brace* **Podcast:** behindthebrace.com/blog
  A podcast hosted by a chiropractor covering various topics about scoliosis to help families live well and stay well.

- **Dr. Derek Lee interview videos:** youtube.com/DerekLee
  Videos of extended discussions with top scoliosis surgeons and other healthcare professionals. An educational resource, these interviews were inspired by his son's own scoliosis journey.

- *Life with Scoliosis* **blog:** lifewithscoliosis.com
  Louise started this blog following her scoliosis fusion surgery in 2010. It is an honest account of life with scoliosis.

- **Scoliosis and Spine Online Learning (SSOL):** scoliosisandspineonlinelearning.com
  Online learning for scoli healthcare professionals. The website includes a video library, webinars, and SSOL certification courses in Lyon and Schroth methods.

- *Tangled in the Curves* **on Instagram:** instagram.com/the_scoliosis_book
  Follow along for continued scoliosis support, resources, information, and fun.

Physical and emotional support

- **Abby Kraai:** abbywiththerods.com
  Abby is a yoga teacher based in Portland, Oregon, specializing in adaptive movement, trauma-informed care, and yoga with scoliosis and spinal fusion. Inspired by her own scoliosis and fusion, she strives to help her students treat their bodies with kindness, and to love their bodies just as they are.

- **Barcelona Scoliosis Physical Therapy School North America:** schroth-barcelonainstitute.com/scoliosis-certified-physical-therapists-usa.html
  Provides a list of Rigo-trained physical therapists across the United States, including contact information.

- **Curvy Girls:** curvygirlsscoliosis.com
  An international support group that empowers teenage girls with scoliosis to come together as they all brave scoliosis.

- **Elisabetta D'Agata, PhD in Psychology (Scoliosis):** psychologyforscoliosis.com
  Elisabetta is a leader in promoting the care of the emotional and psychological effects of scoliosis, knowing firsthand that scoliosis goes beyond the physical. She works with teens and adults with scoliosis. She also works with medical professionals who have scoliosis patients and has published a book detailing the non-physical experience, the impacts, and how to help.

- **Katelyn Carlson:** katelyncarlson.com
  Katelyn offers one-on-one coaching and group workshops to address the mental and emotional challenges included with scoliosis. Having scoliosis herself, she knows this diagnosis goes beyond the physical. She works with scoli teens, parents, and adults with scoliosis who want to come into deeper relationship with their minds, bodies, and spirits, and experience their inherent wholeness.

- **Scolios-us:** bracingforscoliosus.org
  An excellent starting point to gather additional tools and resources. The online platform also offers a mentor program for both bracer and surgery warriors. Kids and teens can connect individually with other people their age who understand what they're experiencing, which can provide some calm in a new world of unknowns.

- **Schroth Method Therapists:** www.schrothmethod.com/contact
  Resources for finding a Schroth therapist for scoliosis treatment, and for becoming Schroth method certified.

- **Strength and Spine LLC:** strengthandspine.com
  Founded by a Schroth physical therapist with scoliosis herself, this company helps people confidently and safely strengthen the body through exercise.

Research and education

- **Back Care Canada:** backcarecanada.ca
  Hosted by the Canadian Spine Society, developed by health professionals to provide advice based on the latest research and professional opinions. It is a good source of information and personal stories.

- **Canada East Spine Center:** canadaeastspine.com
  A multidisciplinary center for spine care, their website has an informative patient education section.

- **Canadian Orthopaedic Foundation:** movepainfree.org
  A Canadian health charity that raises funds to advance orthopaedic research, education, and care. While not scoliosis specific, their website contains information for patient health and surgery.

- **Canadian Spine Society:** spinecanada.ca
  A collaborative organization of spine surgeons and health care professionals with a primary interest in advancing excellence in spine patient care, research and education.

- **International Research Society of Spinal Deformities:** irssd.org
  A forum for presenting and sharing the results of research relating to spinal deformity.

- **International Society on Scoliosis Orthopaedic and Rehabilitation Treatment:** sosort.org
  Dedicated to improving research and the effectiveness of treatment of scoliosis and other structural spine changes.

- **National Association of Spine Specialists:** spine.org
  Provides specific training to healthcare professionals. The website includes consensus and guideline articles from their meetings and workshops.

- **National Scoliosis Foundation:** scoliosis.org
  Provides education to scolis, parents, and healthcare professionals through a variety of resources. The website includes information, an online forum open to the public, and an online store.

- **Scoliosis Association UK:** sauk.org.uk
  Provides advice, support, and information to people and their families affected by scoliosis. They raise awareness of scoliosis among health professionals and the general public.

- **Scoliosis Research Society:** srs.org
  An international society dedicated to research and education in the field of spinal deformities.

- **Setting Scoliosis Straight:** settingscoliosisstraight.org
  A non-profit organization seeking to empower scoli families while supporting scoliosis research. The website offers a variety of patient and parent information in the form of handbooks, videos, and patient stories.

Scoliosis products

- **BackTpack:** backtpack.com
  An ergonomic backpack designed by a physiotherapist, an architect, and their son.

- **Brace Buddies:** bracebuddies.co
  Created by a mother-daughter team who went through scoliosis bracing challenges with few brace undergarments to choose from.

- **Embrace Bags:** embracebags.com
  Cute, sturdy, convenient bags to carry around and protect your back brace.

- **EmBraced in Comfort:** embracedincomfort.com
  Brace-friendly underclothes for both girls and boys.

- **Higgy Bears:** higgybears.com
  With more than 20,000 bears delivered to more than 100 countries, these snuggly friends are helping many patients through tough times. Higgy Bears come with casts, braces, or surgery scars to make scoliosis more "bear-able."

- **Hope's Closet:** hopescloset.com
  Based in the United States by a bracer family who knows what it's like to deal with braces, Hope's Closet provides another option for brace-friendly underclothes.

- **Monkey Butt Powder**: antimonkeybutt.com
  Bracers regularly recommend this product to each other to sooth braces rubbing against sensitive skin.

- **Pillow Pod:** pillowpod.com.au
  A soft full-body pillow, made and shipped in Australia that supports the hips, legs, and shoulders. It can help alleviate aches, pains, and pressures whether you have scoliosis or not.

Endnotes

[1]. "Scoliosis," American Association of Neurological Surgeons, accessed October 31, 2022, https://www.aans.org/Patients/Neurosurgical-Conditions-and-Treatments/Scoliosis.

[2]. American Association of Neurological Surgeons, "Scoliosis."

[3]. "Information and Support," National Scoliosis Foundation, accessed January 3, 2023, https://www.scoliosis.org/info.php.

[4]. "Disability," World Health Organization, accessed October 31, 2022, https://www.who.int/health-topics/disability#tab=tab_1.

[5]. "Scoliosis Braces Market," information by type application, region, forecast till 2030, Straits Research, July 14, 2022, https://straitsresearch.com/report/scoliosis-braces-market.

[6]. Kimberly W McDermott and Lan Liang, "Overview of Operating Room Procedures During Inpatient Stays in US Hospitals, 2018," Healthcare Cost and Utilization Project, Statistical Brief no. 281 (2021), Agency for Healthcare Research and Quality, https://www.hcup-us.ahrq.gov/reports/statbriefs/sb281-Operating-Room-Procedures-During-Hospitalization-2018.jsp.

[7]. American Association of Neurological Surgeons, "Scoliosis."

[8]. American Association of Neurological Surgeons, "Scoliosis."

[9]. "Idiopathic Scoliosis," Boston Children's Hospital, accessed October 25, 2022, https://www.childrenshospital.org/conditions/idiopathic-scoliosis.

[10]. Despina Sapountzi-Krepia, Maria Psychogiou, Darin Peterson, et al., "The Experience of Brace Treatment in Children/Adolescents with Scoliosis," *Scoliosis* 1, no. 8 (2006), National Library of Medicine, https://www.ncbi.nlm.nih.gov/pmc/articles/PMC1481575/.

[11]. American Association of Neurological Surgeons, "Scoliosis."

[12]. "Evaluating Scoliosis – Scoliometer," Scoliosis 3DC, January 26, 2011, https://scoliosis3dc.com/2011/01/26/evaluating-scoliosis-scoliometer/ .

[13]. Hamilton Hall, *A Consultation with the Back Doctor*, McClelland and Stewart, 2003, 34.

[14]. Derek Lee, "Schroth Scoliosis Therapy Everything You Want to Know, Andrea Lebel Interviewed by Dr. Derek Lee," YouTube video, July 7,

2022, https://www.youtube.com/watch?v=DSBdNqgWYkQ&t=5433s&ab_channel=Dr.DerekLee.

15. "Evaluating Scoliosis – Cobb Angle," Scoliosis 3DC, November 15, 2010, https://scoliosis3dc.com/2010/11/15/evaluating-scoliosis-cobb-angle/

16. Jacques H Hacquebord, and Seth S Leopold, "In Brief: The Risser Classification: A Classic Tool for the Clinician Treating Adolescent Idiopathic Scoliosis," *Clinical Orthopaedics and Related Research* 470, no. 8 (2012), https://journals.lww.com/clinorthop/Fulltext/2012/08000/In_Brief__The_Risser_Classification__A_Classic.39.aspx.

17. D'Agata, *Enjoy Life with Idiopathic Scoliosis During Adolescence: Psychology for Professionals of Scoliosis*, Hakabooks, 2019, 59.

18. D'Agata, 52.

19. D'Agata, *Enjoy Life with Idiopathic Scoliosis*, 55.

20. Carol A. Wise, Xiaochong Gao, Scott Shoemaker, et al., "Understanding Genetic Factors in Idiopathic Scoliosis, a Complex Disease of Childhood," *Current Genomics* 9, no. 1 (2008), National Library of Medicine, https://www.ncbi.nlm.nih.gov/pmc/articles/PMC2674301/.

21. Tom Stafford, "Why Can Smells Unlock Forgotten Memories?" *BBC*, March 12, 2012, http://www.bbc.com/future/article/20120312-why-can-smells-unlock-memories.

22. Stafford, "Unlock Forgotten Memories."

23. "EOS Imaging," Hospital for Special Surgery, accessed November 14, 2022, https://www.hss.edu/condition-list_eos-imaging.asp.

24. Derek Lee, "Schroth Scoliosis Therapy."

25. Despina Sapountzi-Krepia et al., "The Experience of Brace Treatment."

26. Sandip P. Tarpada, Matthew T Morris, and Denver A Burton, "Spinal Fusion Surgery: A Historical Perspective," *Journal of Orthopaedics* 14, no. 1 (2016), National Library of Medicine, https://www.ncbi.nlm.nih.gov/pmc/articles/PMC5107724/.

27. Anita Simonds, "Scoliosis and Breathing," Scoliosis Association United Kingdom, accessed November 1, 2022, https://sauk.org.uk/coping-with-scoliosis/scoliosis-and-breathing/.

28. Christa Lehnert, "Scoliosis Exercises for Scoliosis," Schroth Method, accessed November 2, 2022, https://www.schrothmethod.com/scoliosis-exercises.

29. Evin Bozcali, Hanifi Ucpunar, Ahmet Sevencan, et al., "A Retrospective Study of Congenital Cardiac Abnormality Associated with Scoliosis." *Asian Spine Journal* 10, no. 2 (2016), National Library of Medicine, https://www.ncbi.nlm.nih.gov/pmc/articles/PMC4843057/.

30. "Vertebral Body Tethering (VBT)," Boston Children's Hospital, accessed February 17, 2023, https://www.childrenshospital.org/treatments/vertebral-body-tethering.

31. Hall, *A Conversation*, 245.

32. "Sneezing 101 – What Is a Sneeze, Why Do We Sneeze and How to Sneeze Safely," Queensland Health, September 2, 2020, http://www.health.qld.gov.au/news-events/news/sneezing-101-what-why-how-to-sneeze-correctly-safely.

33. "The Water in You: Water and the Human Body," US Geological Survey, May 22, 2019, https://www.usgs.gov/special-topics/water-science-school/science/water-you-water-and-human-body.

34. "Do X-rays and Gamma Rays Cause Cancer?" American Cancer Society, November 10, 2022, https://www.cancer.org/healthy/cancer-causes/radiation-exposure/x-rays-gamma-rays/do-xrays-and-gamma-rays-cause-cancer.html.

35. Adriaan Louw, *Why Do I Hurt? A Patient Book about the Neuroscience of Pain*, Orthopedic Physical Therapy and Rehabilitation Products, 2013, 7.

36. Claudia Katherine, "Pain and Scoliosis – What Is It? How Do We Fix It? Interview with Chronic Pain Specialist Rob Kjemhus," Feel Good Spine (podcast), October 2022, http://www.open.spotify.com/episode/1kjc3YuyNFBnbIcUZr0tUv?si=b1afe926c367429c.

37. Hall, 28.

38. Hall, 27.

39. Hall, 34.

40. Hall, 28.

41. Pradeep Suri, Kathleen W Saunders, and Michael Van Korff, "Prevalence and Characteristics of Flare-ups of Chronic Nonspecific Back Pain in Primary Care: A Telephone Survey," *The Clinical Journal of Pain* 28, no. 7 (2012), https://www.ncbi.nlm.nih.gov/pmc/articles/PMC3414658/.

42. Alex Korb, "Boosting Your Serotonin Activity," Psychology Today, November 17, 2011, https://www.psychologytoday.com/ca/blog/prefrontal-nudity/201111/boosting-your-serotonin-activity.

43. "Sleep Aids: Understand Options Sold without a Prescription," Mayo Clinic, June 8, 2022, https://www.mayoclinic.org/healthy-lifestyle/adult-health/in-depth/sleep-aids/art-20047860.
44. Lee, "Schroth Scoliosis Therapy."
45. Hall, 34.
46. Louw, *Why Do I Hurt*, 16.
47. Louw, 4.
48. Hall, 205.
49. Hall, 207.
50. Beverly Merz, "Healing Through Music," Harvard Health Publishing, November 5, 2015, https://www.health.harvard.edu/blog/healing-through-music-201511058556.
51. "Scoliosis," *Richard III: Discovery and Identification*, University of Leicester, accessed November 22, 2022, https://le.ac.uk/richard-iii/identification/osteology/scoliosis.
52. "General Douglas MacArthur's Scoliosis Story," Strauss Scoliosis Correction, accessed November 8, 2022, https://www.hudsonvalleyscoliosis.com/celebrities-scoliosis/general-douglas-macarthur/.
53. "Empathy," Merriam-Webster, accessed November 7, 2022, https://www.merriam-webster.com/dictionary/empathy.
54. D'Agata, 59.
55. Bill Bryson, *A Short History of Nearly Everything,* Doubleday Canada, 2004, 3.
56. Joelle Hanson-Baiden, "The Debate on Repressed Memories," News Medical, accessed October 31, 2022, https://www.news-medical.net/health/The-Debate-on-Repressed-Memories.aspx.
57. D'Agata, 114.
58. D'Agata, 118.
59. Hall, *A Conversation*, 9, 16.
60. Wise, "Understanding Genetic Factors."
61. Tarpada et al., "Spinal Fusion Surgery."
62. Tarpada et al.
63. Tarpada et al.

64. Tamara Bhandari, "Scoliosis Linked to Essential Mineral," Washington University School of Medicine in St. Louis, October 9, 2018, https://medicine.wustl.edu/news/scoliosis-linked-to-essential-mineral/.

65. Caroline Arbanas, "Scientists Identify First Gene Linked to Scoliosis," The Source, Washington University in St. Louis, June 11, 2007, https://source.wustl.edu/2007/06/scientists-identify-first-gene-linked-to-scoliosis/.

66. "Quasimodo: Hunchback No More," CBS News, June 28, 2002, https://www.cbsnews.com/news/quasimodo-hunchback-no-more/.

67. "Scoliosis and Spine," Scottish Rite for Children, accessed September 29, 2022, https://scottishriteforchildren.org/care-and-treatment/scoliosis-and-spine.

68. D'Agata, 92.

69. "Whether You Believe You Can Do a Thing or Not, You Are Right," Quote Investigator, February 3, 2015, https://quoteinvestigator.com/2015/02/03/you-can/.

Bibliography

Interviews
- Baxter, Peggy (Dr). Personal interview. November 24, 2022.
- Carlson, Katelyn. Personal interview. October 12, 2022.
- Clark, Lily. Personal interview. November 1, 2022.
- Condie, Kyra. Personal interview. October 19, 2022.
- Cunningham, Abby. Personal interview. September 6, 2022.
- D'Agata, Elisabetta. Personal interview. October 18, 2022.
- Dimas, Simone. Personal interview. September 26, 2022.
- Glahn Castille, Megan. Personal interview. October 3, 2022.
- Hale, Emily. "Scoliosis Book Caroline." Received by author October 26, 2022.
- Higginson, Lauren. Personal interview. October 26, 2022.
- Kraai, Abby. Personal interview. December 6, 2022.
- Leonard, Alia. Personal interview. November 2, 2022.
- Lepp, Claudia. Personal interview. October 18, 2022.
- Lynch, Carmen. Personal interview. October 22, 2022.
- Mears, Stacey. "Question about Brace Buddies." Received by author September 9, 2022
- Ouellet, Jean (Dr). Personal interview. December 22, 2022.
- Sherrie, Katherine. Personal interview. October 27, 2022.
- Southard, Katherine. Personal interview. October 27, 2022.

ABC News. "Overcoming the Odds: Tennis Star James Blake." *Good Morning America*, July 30, 2007. https://abcnews.go.com/GMA/story?id=3425892&page=1.

Adobor, Raphael D, Silje Rimeslatten, Harald Steen, et al. "School Screening and Point Prevalence of Adolescent Idiopathic Scoliosis in 4000 Norwegian Children Aged 12 Years." *Scoliosis* 6, no. 23 (2011), BioMed Central. https://scoliosisjournal.biomedcentral.com/articles/10.1186/1748-7161-6-23.

American Academy of Orthopaedic Surgeons. Accessed October 31, 2022. https://www.aaos.org/.

American Association of Neurological Surgeons. "Minimally Invasive Spine Surgery." Accessed August 12, 2022. http://www.aans.org/en/Patients/Neurosurgical-Conditions-and-Treatments/Minimally-Invasive-Spine-Surgery.

American Association of Neurological Surgeons. "Scoliosis." Accessed October 31, 2022. https://www.aans.org/Patients/Neurosurgical-Conditions-and-Treatments/Scoliosis.

American Cancer Society. "Do X-rays and Gamma Rays Cause Cancer?" November 10, 2022. https://www.cancer.org/healthy/cancer-causes/radiation-exposure/x-rays-gamma-rays/do-xrays-and-gamma-rays-cause-cancer.html.

Aquatics International. "Maritza Correia – Crusader." February 1, 2007. https://www.aquaticsintl.com/awards/maritza-correia-crusader_o.

Arbanas, Caroline. "Scientists Identify First Gene Linked to Scoliosis." *The Source*, Washington University in St. Louis, June 11, 2007. http://source.wustl.edu/2007/06/scientists-identify-first-gene-linked-to-scoliosis.

Arnold, Amanda. "Laura Dern Is So Good at Sitting." *The Cut*, December 19, 2019, https://www.thecut.com/2019/12/laura-dern-sitting-icon.html.

Attias, Daniel, director. "Underage Drinking: A National Concern." *It's Always Sunny in Philadelphia*, season 1, episode 3, FX, August 16, 2005.

Berdishevsky, Hagit, Victoria Ashley Lebel, Josette Bettany-Saltikov, et al. "Physiotherapy Scoliosis-Specific Exercises – A Comprehensive Review of Seven Major Schools." *Scoliosis* 11, no. 20 (2016), BioMed Central. https://scoliosisjournal.biomedcentral.com/articles/10.1186/s13013-016-0076-9.

Bhandari, Tamara. "Scoliosis Linked to Essential Mineral." Washington University School of Medicine in St. Louis, October 9, 2018. https://medicine.wustl.edu/news/scoliosis-linked-to-essential-mineral/.

Biggers, Larissa. "EOS Imaging Reduces Radiation Exposure for Children with Scoliosis." *Duke Health* (blog), November 2, 2021. http://www.dukehealth.org/blog/eos-imaging-reduces-radiation-exposure-children-scoliosis.

Binner, Andrew. "Five things to know about David Popovici: The Romanian swimmer destined for greatness." *Olympics.com,* June 22, 2022. *https*://olympics.com/en/news/five-facts-david-popovici-swimming-world-champion.

Biography. "Yo-Yo Ma." April 2, 2014, updated May 19, 2021. https://www.biography.com/musician/yo-yo-ma.

Boland, Katie. "This week in Inspiring Women: Anne Murray." *She Does the City* (blog). October 21, 2010. https://www.shedoesthecity.com/this_week_in_inspiring_women_anne_murray/.

Boston Children's Hospital. "Idiopathic Scoliosis." Accessed October 25, 2022. https://www.childrenshospital.org/conditions/idiopathic-scoliosis.

Boston Children's Hospital. "Vertebral Body Tethering (VBT)." Accessed February 17, 2023. https://www.childrenshospital.org/treatments/vertebral-body-tethering.

Bozcali, Evin, Hanifi Ucpunar, Ahmet Sevencan, et al. "A Retrospective Study of Congenital Cardiac Abnormality Associated with Scoliosis." *Asian Spine Journal* 10, no. 2 (2016), National Library of Medicine. https://www.ncbi.nlm.nih.gov/pmc/articles/PMC4843057/.

Brace Buddies. Accessed August 12, 2022. http://www.bracebuddies.co.

Broeren, Jessa. "They Have Scoliosis!? Famous and Influential People That You Never Knew Had Scoliosis." *The Girl with the Spine Thing* (blog), February 21, 2019. https://www.girlwiththespinething.com/single-post/2019/02/21/they-have-scoliosis-famous-and-influential-people-that-you-never-knew-had-scoliosis.

Bryson, Bill. *A Short History of Nearly Everything.* Doubleday Canada, 2004.

CBS News. "Quasimodo: Hunchback No More." June 28, 2002, https://www.cbsnews.com/news/quasimodo-hunchback-no-more/.

Chetia, Aklanta. "Usain Bolt Defeated a Career-Threatening Medical Condition to Become the World's Fastest Man." EssentiallySports, June 1, 2022. https://www.essentiallysports.com/us-sports-news-track-and-field-news-usain-bolt-defeated-a-career-threatening-medical-condition-to-become-the-worlds-fastest-man/.

Children's Healthcare of Atlanta. "Do You Think Your Child's Spine Is Curved? She Might Have Scoliosis." Accessed October 31, 2022. https://www.choa.org/parent-resources/orthopedics/signs-of-scoliosis-in-children.

Columbia Neurosurgery. "Instrumented Spinal Fusion." Columbia University Irving Medical Center. Accessed August 6, 2022. https://www.neurosurgery.columbia.edu/patient-care/treatments/instrumented-spinal-fusion.

Cooke, Pam, Jansen Yee, Ron Hughart, et al., directors. "Chimdale." *American Dad!* season 4, episode 8, Fox, January 25, 2009.

Côté, Pierre, B G Kreitz, J David Cassidy, et al. "A Study of the Diagnostic Accuracy and Reliability of the Scoliometer and Adam's Forward Bend Test." *Spine* 23, no. 7 (1998), PubMed. https://pubmed.ncbi.nlm.nih.gov/9563110/.

Cullity, Mike. "Golfer Stacy Lewis: Scoliosis Can't Stop Me." ESPN, June 1, 2012. https://www.espn.com/blog/high-school/girl/post/_/id/2218/stacy-lewis-scoliosis-made-me-who-i-am.

Curvy Girls. "Got Scoliosis? You're Not Alone!" 2022. http://www.curvygirlsscoliosis.com.

Czaprowski, Dariusz, Tomasz Kotwicki, Paulina Pawlowska, et al. "Joint Hypermobility in Children with Idiopathic Scoliosis: SOSORT Award 2011 Winner." *Scoliosis* 6, no. 22 (2011), BioMed Central. https://scoliosisjournal.biomedcentral.com/articles/10.1186/1748-7161-6-22.

Daily Hawker. "Rene Russo: 8 Facts about the Lethal Weapon Actress That Fans Will Love!" October 13, 2020. https://www.dailyhawker.ca/rene-russo/.

D'Agata, Elisabetta. *Enjoy Life with Idiopathic Scoliosis During Adolescence: Psychology for Professionals of Scoliosis*. Hakabooks, 2019.

Dietz, Mandy. "The Wait and See Mentality in Scoliosis." *Behind the Brace Podcast*, September 7, 2021. http://behindthebrace.com/2021/09/07/5-the-wait-and-see-mentality-in-scoliosis/.

Disc of Louisiana. "Kurt Cobain says scoliosis got worse from playing the guitar." June 23, 2021. https://geauxspine.com/kurt-cobain-says-scoliosis-got-worse-from-playing-the-guitar/

Disc Spine Institute. "Advances in Scoliosis Treatment Are Changing Lives." *Back Stories*, July 5, 2017. https://www.discspine.com/back-stories/new-advancements-scoliosis-treatment.

Gao, Xiaochong, Derek Gordon, Dongping Zhang, et al. "CHD7 Gene Polymorphisms Are Associated with Susceptibility to Idiopathic Scoliosis." *American Journal of Human Genetics* 80, no. 5 (2007): 957–65, National Library of Medicine. https://pubmed.ncbi.nlm.nih.gov/17436250/.

Gates, Tucker, director. "The Apartment." *Brooklyn Nine-Nine*, season 1, episode 18, Fox, February 25, 2014.

Gerber, Alyson. *Braced*. New York: Arthur A. Levine Books, 2017.

Grillo. "Coming Out of My Plastic Shell." *Lenny*, March 30, 2018. http://www.lennyletter.com/story/coming-out-of-my-plastic-shell.

Grimes, Kelly. "What Do We Know about What Causes Adolescent Idiopathic Scoliosis." Scolios-us, February 25, 2021. http://www.bracing-forscoliosus.org/what-causes-adolescent-idiopathic-scoliosis.

Grivas, Theodoros B, R Geoffrey Burwell, Constantinos Mihas, et al. "Relatively Lower Body Mass Index Is Associated with an Excess of Severe Truncal Asymmetry in Healthy Adolescents: Do White Adipose Tissue, Leptin, Hypothalamus and Sympathetic Nervous System Influence Truncal Growth Asymmetry?" *Scoliosis* 4, no. 13 (2009), BioMed Central. https://scoliosisjournal.biomedcentral.com/articles/10.1186/1748-7161-4-13.

Guglielmi, Jodi. "Isabella Rossellini Recalls Mom Ingrid Bergman Quitting Career to Be at Her Bedside for Two Years During Illness." People, December 4, 2015. https://people.com/movies/isabella-rossellini-recalls-ingrid-bergman-quitting-acting-to-be-at-her-bedside/.

Hacquebord, Jacques H, and Seth S Leopold. "In Brief: The Risser Classification: A Classic Tool for the Clinician Treating Adolescent Idiopathic Scoliosis." *Clinical Orthopaedics and Related Research* 470, no. 8 (2012). https://journals.lww.com/clinorthop/Fulltext/2012/08000/In_Brief__The_Risser_Classification__A_Classic.39.aspx.

Hall, Hamilton. *A Consultation with the Back Doctor*. McClelland and Stewart, 2003.

Hanson-Baiden, Joelle. "The Debate on Repressed Memories." News Medical. Accessed October 31, 2022. https://www.news-medical.net/health/The-Debate-on-Repressed-Memories.aspx.

Hawes, Martha C. *Scoliosis and the Human Spine*. n.p.: Martha C Hawes, 2002.

Health Guide. "Famous People with Scoliosis." July 12, 2022. https://healthguidenet.com/conditions/famous-people-with-scoliosis/.

Health Research Funding. "Famous People with Scoliosis." Accessed February 19, 2023. https://healthresearchfunding.org/famous-people-scoliosis/.

Hohman, Maura. "Princess Eugenie Just Shared X-Rays from Her Childhood Scoliosis Surgery for the First Time." People, July 2, 2018. https://people.com/royals/princess-eugenie-shares-x-rays-scoliosis-surgery/.

Hospital for Special Surgery. "EOS Imaging." Accessed November 14, 2022. https://www.hss.edu/condition-list_eos-imaging.asp.

Hughes, John, director. *Sixteen Candles*. Universal Pictures, 1984.

Iles, Brian, Dominic Bianchi, and James Purdum, directors. "The Dating Game." *Family Guy*, season 15, episode 14, Fox, March 5, 2017.

IMDb. Accessed November 18, 2022. https://www.imdb.com/.

International Society on Scoliosis Orthopaedic and Rehabilitation Treatment. Accessed July 2, 2022. http://www.sosort.org.

Jann, Michael Patrick, director. "Magazine Profile." *Superstore*, season 1, episode 2, NBC, November 30, 2015.

Jasiewicz, Barbara, Tomasz Potaczek, Maciej Tesiorowski, et al. "Spine Deformities in Patients with Ehlers-Danlos Syndrome, Type IV – Late Results of Surgical Treatment." *Scoliosis* 5, no. 26 (2010), BioMed Central. https://scoliosisjournal.biomedcentral.com/articles/10.1186/1748-7161-5-26.

Jeon, Kyoungkyu, and Dong-il Kim. "The Association Between Low Body Weight and Scoliosis Among Korean Elementary School Students." *International Journal of Environmental Research and Public Health* 15, no. 12 (2018): 2613, National Library of Medicine. https://www.ncbi.nlm.nih.gov/pmc/articles/PMC6313767/.

Johns Hopkins Medicine. "Scoliosis." Accessed November 4, 2022. https://www.hopkinsmedicine.org/health/conditions-and-diseases/scoliosis.

Kanner, Ellie, director. "Depth Perception." *Greek*, season 1, episode 9, ABC Family, September 3, 2007.

Karas, Jay, director. "Cherry Picker." *The Mighty Ducks: Game Changers*, season 1, episode 5, Goldsmith Yuspa Productions, Brillstein Entertainment Partners, ABC Signature, April 23, 2021.

Katherine, Claudia. "Pain and Scoliosis – What Is It? How Do We Fix It? Interview with Chronic Pain Specialist Rob Kjemhus." Feel Good Spine (podcast), October 31, 2022. http://www.open.spotify.com/episode/1kjc3YuyNFBnbIcUZr0tUv?si=b1afe926c367429c.

Korb, Alex. "Boosting Your Serotonin Activity." Psychology Today, November 17, 2011, https://www.psychologytoday.com/ca/blog/prefrontal-nudity/201111/boosting-your-serotonin-activity.

Ledbetter, Carly. "Princess Eugenie's Low-Backed Wedding Dress Shows off Scoliosis Scars." *HuffPost*, October 12, 2018. https://www.huffpost.com/entry/princess-eugenie-wedding-dress_n_5bbf98ebe4b01a01d688a793?ncid=engmodushpmg00000003&fbclid=IwAR3O_47e1h6D5M5xMcIopLlmlWON_Fkp1sQsl6ZJLnbca2eDEt_akkW_LcU.

Lee, Derek. "Schroth Scoliosis Therapy Everything You Want to Know, Andrea Lebel Interviewed by Dr. Derek Lee." YouTube video, July 7, 2022. https://www.youtube.com/watch?v=DSBdNqgWYkQ&t=5433s&ab_channel=Dr.DerekLee.

Lee, Derek. "Scoliosis Bracing Everything You Want to Know, Luke Stikeleather Interviewed by Dr. Derek Lee." YouTube video, June 29, 2020. https://www.youtube.com/watch?v=DRqFhgn1T8I&ab_channel=Dr.DerekLee.

Lee, Jeanette. "Champion Pool Player Turns Pain into Will to Win." *The Human Factor with Dr. Sanjay Gupta*, CNN Health, March 31, 2016. https://www.cnn.com/2016/03/31/health/turning-points-jeanette-lee-op-ed-article.

Levy, Benjamin J., Shulz, Jacob F., Fornari, Eric D., et al. "Complications Associated with Surgical Repair of Syndromic Scoliosis." *Scoliosis* 10, no. 14 (2015), BioMed Central. https://scoliosisjournal.biomedcentral.com/articles/10.1186/s13013-015-0035-x.

Lewis, Stacy. "Scoliosis Hasn't Stopped Top Female Golfer." CNN Health, June 6, 2013. https://edition.cnn.com/2013/06/06/health/human-factor-lewis/index.html.

Lopez, Alex Garcia, director. "Betrayer Moon." *The Witcher*, season 1, episode 3, Little Schmidt Productions, Hivemind, Platige Image, December 20, 2019.

Louw, Adriaan. *Why Do I Hurt? A Patient Book about the Neuroscience of Pain*. Orthopedic Physical Therapy and Rehabilitation Products, 2013.

Lutton, Phil. "Standing Tall: Jessica Ashwood Is Finally on the Straight and Narrow." *The Sydney Morning Herald*, May 25, 2019. https://www.smh.com.au/sport/swimming/standing-tall-jessica-ashwood-is-finally-on-the-straight-and-narrow-20190515-p51nqs.html.

Malfair, David, Anne K Flemming, Marcel F Dvorak, et al. "Radiographic Evaluation of Scoliosis: Review." *American Journal of Roentgenology* 194, no. 3_supplement (2010). https://www.ajronline.org/doi/10.2214/AJR.07.7145.

Masters, Samantha. "Rita Simons 'Desperate for Operation' as Scoliosis Worsens 'I'm in a Whole World of Pain.'" Express, February 24, 2021. https://www.express.co.uk/celebrity-news/1402038/rita-simons-scoliosis-spine-condition-health-eastenders-news-latest-update.

Mayo Clinic. "Sleep Aids: Understand Options Sold without a Prescription." June 8, 2022. https://www.mayoclinic.org/healthy-lifestyle/adult-health/in-depth/sleep-aids/art-20047860.

McAfee, Paul. "Types of Scoliosis Braces." Spine-health, December 8, 2016. https://www.spine-health.com/conditions/scoliosis/types-scoliosis-braces.

McDermott, Julianna. "Former Model with Scoliosis, Ayesha Jones, Turns to Photography to Challenge Beauty Ideals." HuffPost, July 15, 2015. https://www.huffpost.com/archive/ca/entry/former-model-with-scoliosis-ayesha-jones-turns-to-photography_n_7796262.

McDermott, Kimberly W, and Lan Liang. "Overview of Operating Room Procedures During Inpatient Stays in US Hospitals, 2018." Healthcare Cost and Utilization Project, Statistical Brief no. 281 (2021), Agency for Healthcare Research and Quality. https://www.hcup-us.ahrq.gov/reports/statbriefs/sb281-Operating-Room-Procedures-During-Hospitalization-2018.jsp.

Melman, Jeff, director. "Thank God for Scoliosis." *Two and a Half Men*, season 6, episode 12, CBS, January 12, 2009.

Mendoza, Linda, director. "Return to Skyfire." *Brooklyn Nine-Nine*, season 5, episode 8, Fox, November 28, 2017.

Merriam-Webster. "Empathy." Accessed November 7, 2022. https://www.merriam-webster.com/dictionary/empathy.

Merz, Beverly. "Healing Through Music." Harvard Health Publishing, November 5, 2015. https://www.health.harvard.edu/blog/healing-through-music-201511058556.

Mirkin, David, director. *Romy and Michele's High School Reunion*. Touchstone Pictures, 1997.

Nahas, Aili. "Giuliana Rancic: 'I Was Called Ugly My Entire Life.'" People, December 2, 2020. https://people.com/celebrity/giuliana-rancic-talks-scoliosis-weight-being-called-ugly/.

National Scoliosis Foundation. Accessed September 21, 2022. http://www.scoliosis.org.

NPR. "Plenty of 'Big Love' for HBO Star Chloe Sevigny." Interview by Terry Gross. *Fresh Air,* March 2, 2010. https://www.npr.org/transcripts/124198338.

Paharia, Pooja Toshniwal. "What is the Nervous System?" News Medical, September 4, 2022. https://www.news-medical.net/health/What-is-the-Nervous-System.aspx.

Park, Michael Y. "Rebecca Romijn Hopes to Be 'Lucky' and Have Kids." People, July 16, 2008. https://people.com/celebrity/rebecca-romijn-hopes-to-be-lucky-and-have-kids/.

Polley, Sarah. "Caught Through the Looking Glass: Sarah Polley on Grief, Girlhood, and Scoliosis." *Literary Hub*, March 2, 2022. https://lithub.com/caught-through-the-looking-glass-sarah-polley-on-grief-girlhood-and-scoliosis/.

Probst, Jeff, director. *Kiss Me*. MysticArt Pictures, 2014.

PT Direct. "Nervous System: Anatomy and Function." Accessed October 2022. https://www.ptdirect.com/training-design/anatomy-and-physiology/the-nervous-system-2013-anatomy-and-function.

Qiu, Yong, Xu Sun, Xusheng Qiu, et al. "Decreased Circulating Leptin Level and Its Association with Body and Bone Mass in Girls with Adolescent Idiopathic Scoliosis." *Spine* 32, no. 24 (2007): 2703–2710, National Library of Medicine. https://pubmed.ncbi.nlm.nih.gov/18007248/.

Quote Investigator. "Whether You Believe You Can Do a Thing or Not, You Are Right." February 3, 2015, https://quoteinvestigator.com/2015/02/03/you-can/.

Queensland Health. "Sneezing 101 – What Is a Sneeze, Why Do We Sneeze and How to Sneeze Safely." September 2, 2020. https://www.health.qld.gov.au/news-events/news/sneezing-101-what-why-how-to-sneeze-correctly-safely.

Sapountzi-Krepia, Despina, Maria Psychogiou, Darin Peterson, et al. "The Experience of Brace Treatment in Children/Adolescents with Scoliosis." *Scoliosis* 1, no. 8 (2006), National Library of Medicine. https://www.ncbi.nlm.nih.gov/pmc/articles/PMC1481575/.

Savage, Fred, director. "The Aluminum Monster vs. Fatty Magoo." *It's Always Sunny in Philadelphia*, season 3, episode 5, FX, September 27, 2007.

Schad, Tom. "US Olympic Sport Climber Kyra Condie Not Slowed after 10 Fused Vertebrae in Her Spine." USA Today, August 3, 2021. http://www.usatoday.com/story/sports/olympics/2021/08/03/

tokyo-olympics-sport-climber-kyra-condie-not-slowed-spinal-fusion-surgery/8000168002/.

Scheerer, Mark. "Country Music Finds Teen Singer Jessica Andrews." CNN, April 15, 1999. http://www.cnn.com/SHOWBIZ/Music/9904/15/jessica.andrews/.

Schroth Method. "How the Schroth Method Works." Accessed July 2, 2022. http://www.schrothmethod.com/about-schroth-method.

Schroth Method. "Schroth Exercises for Scoliosis." Accessed November 2, 2022. https://www.schrothmethod.com/scoliosis-exercises.

Scoliosis 3DC. "Evaluating Scoliosis – Cobb Angle." November 15, 2010. https://scoliosis3dc.com/2010/11/15/evaluating-scoliosis-cobb-angle/.

Scoliosis 3DC. "Evaluating Scoliosis – Scoliometer." January 26, 2011. https://scoliosis3dc.com/2011/01/26/evaluating-scoliosis-scoliometer/.

Scoliosis 3DC. "Scoliosis Angle – What is the Difference Between the Cobb Angle and Scoliometer Measurement?" February 22, 2016. https://scoliosis3dc.com/2016/02/22/scoliosis-angle-difference-between-cobb-angle-and-scoliometer/.

Scoliosis and Spine Online Learning. Accessed August 12, 2022. http://www.scoliosisandspineonlinelearning.com.

Scoliosis Research Society. "Martha's Story: Walking Straight Down the Runway." *Patients and Families*. Accessed September 21, 2022. https://www.srs.org/patients-and-families/patient-stories/martha.

Scolios-us. "Scolios-us: Putting the 'Us' in Scoliosis." Accessed September 2022. http://www.bracingforscoliosus.org.

Scottish Rite for Children. "Scoliosis and Spine." Accessed October 29, 2022. http://www.scottishriteforchildren.org/care-and-treatment/scoliosis-and-spine.

Setting Scoliosis Straight. "2021 Annual Report." Accessed October 24, 2022. https://www.settingscoliosisstraight.org/annual-report/.

Shakman, Matt, director. "Dennis and Dee's Mom Is Dead." *It's Always Sunny in Philadelphia*, season 3, episode 3, FX, September 20, 2007.

Shakman, Matt, director. "The High School Reunion." *It's Always Sunny in Philadelphia*, season 7, episode 12, FX, December 8, 2011.

Shakman, Matt, director. "The High School Reunion Part 2: The Gang's Revenge." *It's Always Sunny in Philadelphia*, season 7, episode 13, FX, December 15, 2011.

Shriners Children's. "MAGEC System – MAGnetic Expansion Control Spinal Bracing and Distraction System." Accessed August 12, 2022. https://www.shrinerschildrens.org/en/pediatric-care/magec-system.

Shriners Children's. "Scoliosis." Accessed November 18, 2022. https://www.shrinerschildrens.org/en/pediatric-care/scoliosis.

Simonds, Anita. "Scoliosis and Breathing." Scoliosis Association United Kingdom. Accessed November 1, 2022. https://sauk.org.uk/coping-with-scoliosis/scoliosis-and-breathing/.

Simone Fortier. "Stretch the Curve Out of Scoliosis." June 13, 2017. https://www.simonefortier.com/blog/health-wellness/stretch-the-curve-out-of-scoliosis/.

Sorkin, Aaron, director. *Molly's Game*. STX Entertainment, Huayi Brothers Pictures, The Mark Gordon Company, Pascal Pictures, Entertainment One, Sierra/Affinity, 2017.

SpineCor. Accessed September 21,2022. https://www.spinecor.com/.

Stafford, Tom. "Why Can Smells Unlock Forgotten Memories?" BBC, March 12, 2012. https://www.bbc.com/future/article/20120312-why-can-smells-unlock-memories.

Straits Research. "Scoliosis Braces Market." Information by type application, region, forecast till 2030. July 14, 2022. https://straitsresearch.com/report/scoliosis-braces-market.

Strauss Scoliosis Correction. "Celebrities with Scoliosis." Hudson Valley Scoliosis. Accessed September 21, 2022. https://www.hudsonvalleyscoliosis.com/celebrities-scoliosis/celebrities/.

Strauss Scoliosis Correction. "Elizabeth Taylor's Scoliosis Story." Hudson Valley Scoliosis. Accessed November 22, 2022. https://www.hudsonvalleyscoliosis.com/celebrities-scoliosis/elizabeth-taylor/.

Strauss Scoliosis Correction. "General Douglas MacArthur's Scoliosis Story." Hudson Valley Scoliosis. Accessed November 8, 2022. https://www.hudsonvalleyscoliosis.com/celebrities-scoliosis/general-douglas-macarthur/.

Suri, Pradeep, Kathleen W Saunders, and Michael Van Korff. "Prevalence and Characteristics of Flare-ups of Chronic Non-specific Back Pain in Primary Care: A Telephone Survey." *Clinical Journal of Pain* 28, no. 7 (2012), National Library of Medicine. https://www.ncbi.nlm.nih.gov/pmc/articles/PMC3414658/.

Tarpada, Sandip P, Matthew T Morris, and Denver A Burton. "Spinal Fusion Surgery: A Historical Perspective." *Journal of Orthopaedics* 14, no. 1 (2016), National Library of Medicine. https://www.ncbi.nlm.nih.gov/pmc/articles/PMC5107724/.

Théroux, Jean, Sylvie Le May, Carole Fortin, et al. "Prevalence and Management of Back Pain in Adolescent Idiopathic Scoliosis Patients: A Retrospective Study." *Pain Research and Management* 20, no. 3 (May–June 2015): 153–7, National Library of Medicine. https://www.ncbi.nlm.nih.gov/pmc/articles/PMC4447159/.

Truumees, David, Ashley Duncan, Eric Kano Mayer, et al. "Social Media as a New Source of Medical Information and Support: Analysis of Scoliosis-Specific Information." *Spine Deformity* 9, no. 5 (2021): 1241–45, National Library of Medicine. https://pubmed.ncbi.nlm.nih.gov/33826124/.

University of Leicester. "Scoliosis." *Richard III: Discovery and Identification.* Accessed November 22, 2022. https://le.ac.uk/richard-iii/identification/osteology/scoliosis.

US Geological Survey. "The Water in You: Water and the Human Body." May 22, 2019. https://www.usgs.gov/special-topics/water-science-school/science/water-you-water-and-human-body.

Wang, Jing, Jin Zhang, Rui Xu, et al. "Measurement of Scoliosis Cobb Angle by End Vertebra Tilt Angle Method." *Journal of Orthopaedic Surgery and Research* 13, no. 223 (2018), BioMed Central. https://josr-online.biomedcentral.com/articles/10.1186/s13018-018-0928-5.

Watanabe, Kota, Takehiro Michikawa, Ikuho Yonezawa, et al. "Physical Activities and Lifestyle Factors Related to Adolescent Idiopathic Scoliosis." *The Journal of Bone and Joint Surgery* 99, no. 4 (2017): 284–94. https://journals.lww.com/jbjsjournal/Abstract/2017/02150/Physical_Activities_and_Lifestyle_Factors_Related.2.aspx.

Weiss, Hans-Rudolph. "The Method of Katharina Schroth – History, Principles and Current Development." *Scoliosis* 6, no. 17 (2011), BioMed Central. https://scoliosisjournal.biomedcentral.com/articles/10.1186/1748-7161-6-17.

Wiedemann, Elettra. "Model Elettra Wiedemann Opens up about Her Teenage Struggle with Scoliosis." *Teen Vogue*, August 6, 2013. https://www.teenvogue.com/story/elettra-wiedemann-struggle-with-scoliosis.

Wise, Carol A, Xiaochong Gao, Scott Shoemaker, et al. "Understanding Genetic Factors in Idiopathic Scoliosis, a Complex Disease of Childhood." *Current Genomics* 9, no. 1 (2008), National Library of Medicine. https://www.ncbi.nlm.nih.gov/pmc/articles/PMC2674301/.

Wolf, Fred, director. *The House Bunny*. Columbia Pictures, Relativity Media, Happy Madison Productions, 2008.

World Health Organization. "Disability and health." Accessed October 31, 2022. https://www.who.int/health-topics/disability#tab=tab_1.

Yaitanes, Greg, director. "Six Days (Part 1)." *Grey's Anatomy*, season 3, episode 11, ABC, January 11, 2007.

Yaitanes, Greg, director. "Six Days (Part 2)." *Grey's Anatomy*, season 3, episode 12, ABC, January 18, 2007.

Yeramosu, Teja, Calista L Dominy, Varun Arvind, et al. "Scoliosis Surgery: A Social Media Analysis of Content, Tone, and Perspective." *Journal of the American Academy of Orthopaedic Surgeons* 31, no. 1 (2023), National Library of Medicine. https://pubmed.ncbi.nlm.nih.gov/36162006/.

Milton Keynes UK
Ingram Content Group UK Ltd.
UKHW041427010824
1122UKWH00050B/359